A World Growing Old

The Coming Health Care Challenges

Hastings Center Studies in Ethics

A SERIES EDITED BY

Mark J. Hanson and Daniel Callahan

Established in 1969, The Hastings Center, located in Briarcliff Manor, New York, is an independent, nonprofit, and nonpartisan research organization that examines ethical issues in medicine and the life sciences. The work of the Center is mainly carried out through research projects, the publication of the *Hastings Center Report* and *IRB: A Review of Human Subjects Research,* and numerous workshops, conferences, lectures, and consultations. The *Hastings Center Studies in Ethics* is a series intended to bring the ongoing research work of The Hastings Center to a wider audience.

R

A World Growing Old
The Coming Health Care Challenges

EDITED BY
Daniel Callahan
Ruud H. J. ter Meulen
Eva Topinková

GEORGETOWN UNIVERSITY PRESS / WASHINGTON, D.C.

Georgetown University Press, Washington, D.C. 20007
© 1995 by Georgetown University Press. All rights reserved.
Printed in the United States of America
10 9 8 7 6 5 4 3 2   1995
THIS VOLUME IS PRINTED ON ACID-FREE ∞ OFFSET BOOK PAPER

Library of Congress Cataloging-in-Publication Data
A world growing old : the coming health care challenges / edited by
  Daniel Callahan, Ruud H. J. ter Meulen, Eva Topinková.
      p.   cm.——(Hastings Center studies in ethics)
      ISBN 0-87840-591-7
      1. Aged—Medical care—Social aspects.   2. Aged—Medical care—
  Government policy.   3. Aged—Medical care—Moral and ethical
  aspects.   I. Callahan, Daniel, 1930–   .   II. Meulen, R. H. J. ter
  (Ruud H. J.), 1952–   .   III. Topinková, Eva.   IV. Series.
  RA564.8.W69   1995
  362.1'9897—dc20   95-6447

Contents

Preface

This book is the outcome of a two-year research project entitled "Care for the Elderly: Goals, Resources, Priorities," organized jointly by The Institute for Bioethics, Maastricht, the Netherlands, and The Hastings Center, Briarcliff Manor, N.Y., USA. We would like to acknowledge the generous financial support of the following organizations:

- The Commission of the European Communities, Brussels, Belgium
- Stichting Fondsenwervingsacties Volksgezondheid, The Hague, the Netherlands
- Stichting Algemene Loterij Nederland, The Hague, the Netherlands
- The Pettus-Crowe Foundation, Washington, D.C., USA

Finally, the editors would like to thank Mark J. Hanson of The Hastings Center and the editors of the *Hastings Center Report* for their assistance in making this collection possible. We would also like to thank Anneke van den Berg Jeths of the National Institute for Public Health and Environmental Care, the Netherlands, and Carine van Wanseele, of the Vrije Universiteit, Brussels, Belgium, for their great assistance to us in our research work.

The chapter "What Do We Owe the Elderly? Allocating Social and Health Care Resources" originally appeared as a special supplement in the *Hastings Center Report* 24, no. 2 (1994): S4-S12.

Daniel Callahan, Ruud H. J. ter Meulen, and
Eva Topinková

Introduction

It is hardly news any longer that health care for the elderly looms as one of the most daunting problems in the decades ahead. Demographic projections in every developed country point to a great increase in the number and proportion of the elderly, particularly after 2005, together with a corresponding decline in the number and proportion of younger people—those who will have financial and social responsibility for the old. The projected increase in the elderly is particularly notable for those over the age of eighty-five.

While a majority of elderly people, particularly those in their late sixties and seventies, are healthy and vigorous, many are not, and by their eighties more and more will be burdened by some degree of chronic illness or disability or both. The scarcity of resources for institutional and home care is a vexing, painful problem for many countries already and may only get worse in the future. The growing needs of the elderly come, unfortunately, at a time when the governments of almost all developed countries are under great budgetary pressures, exacerbated all the more by the increase in more successful—but often more costly—high-technology and acute-care medical interventions with the old.

Though most governments have not been indifferent to these trends, little serious planning or even serious discussion about the future has taken place. The issue of allocation of resources to the elderly is, almost everywhere, a difficult and delicate subject. While some nations have politically active groups of elderly people speaking effectively for themselves, many others do not. And while many countries are trying to think about the health care needs of the elderly, the pressures to hold down costs seem to make few options available to them.

To address some of these problems, The Hastings Center and The Institute for Bioethics in Maastricht, the Netherlands, jointly organized an international project on resource allocation and the elderly. Representatives from some eight countries took part: Sweden, Belgium, Germany, the United Kingdom, the Czech Republic, Hungary, the Netherlands, and the United States. It was a lively and interesting group, different in perspectives, disciplinary backgrounds, and cultures but sharing a desire to bring to greater public and professional attention the developing problems in health care for the elderly.

The first task of the project participants was to find a helpful way to formulate the issues, and particularly to put the health care problems in the most revealing context. The group settled on five main areas of concern:

- *The meaning and significance of old age.* How are we in modern societies to understand the place of aging in the life cycle, the significance of old age in society, and the meaning the elderly themselves bring to their situation?

- *The goals of medicine and health care for the elderly.* Health care for the elderly has undergone great changes in recent decades, in particular opening up new possibilities for improved health: how should medicine now formulate its goals in health care for the elderly?

- *Balancing the needs of the young and old.* Since it will be the young who will have to bear the health care costs of the old, what may the old reasonably demand, and what ought the young reasonably be expected to do for them?

- *Resource allocation and social priorities.* Every health care system now faces financial strain. How should societies think about allocating resources to the old, and if limits are necessary, what is the fairest way of setting them?

- *Families, society, women, and long-term care.* How far can families be expected to go to provide care for their elderly members, and how, in the future, can less unfair pressure be placed on women to provide informal care?

Each of these five general issues proved difficult, some because they raise profound moral problems and others because, though the moral problems seemed less daunting, the practical issues may be even more so. It is important to recognize that the Western European countries are now reducing their traditional emphasis on the welfare state and are working to privatize parts of their health care systems. As in the United States, the public is resisting higher taxes. In the Central European countries, enormous reform efforts are underway, but the shortage of money is even more severe. These changes in the economic viability of current health care systems come at a bad moment, when the need and public demand for good health care for the elderly will continue to rise.

The chapters in this collection have been written by project participants and others commissioned to cover the main topics of the project. The book begins with Mark J. Hanson's review of the project's country reports, documents written by representatives from countries participating in the research work.

This chapter helps set the empirical context for the other essays by summarizing under broad themes how different countries are facing the growing challenges of caring for their elderly. Utilizing the comparative categories of demographics, developments in medical technology, the structure of health care systems, economics, and the elderly's social status, Hanson's report reveals a fair amount of common ground among countries regarding problems under each of these categories, despite quite different social and economic backgrounds.

The next three chapters lay the foundation for the rest of the book by addressing fundamental issues for any consideration of health care problems for the elderly: the meaning of old age and medicine's goals in response to it. Harry R. Moody argues that any decisions about health care allocation for the elderly will rely on questions of what a society thinks old age means. He provides four scenarios for the future that help define four approaches to the meaning of old age.

Daniel Callahan takes a somewhat different approach to essentially the same set of issues. He develops two models of the goals of medicine in response to aging. "Progressive incrementalism" is characterized by a steady pushing of the limits of morbidity and mortality and is essentially dedicated to unlimited progress in the long run. "Life cycle traditionalism" is skeptical of this endeavor and sets limits on it through appeals to the biological rhythm of the life cycle. Callahan concludes with arguments in favor of the latter approach.

Paul van Tongeren explores philosophically an issue raised by both Moody and Callahan, namely, the desire of persons to extend their lives. He argues that consideration of this desire should lead us not to provide resources toward the goal of life extension, but, rather, toward that which promotes reflection on the meaning of life and why we resist death.

Against the background of these more philosophical issues, the next two chapters begin the work of considering some of the more practical concerns of health care resource allocation for the elderly, beginning with the difficult job of projecting the actual extent of future resource scarcity. Anneke van den Berg Jeths and Mats Thorslund draw on research from the Netherlands and Sweden to explore trends in resource utilization by the elderly as well as government responses. While presenting various difficulties in making long-term projections, they concede that predictable demographic changes will bring an increased demand for services by the elderly and that consideration of priority setting for health care resource allocation can and must begin today.

Reiner Leidl's essay examines specifically the effects of population aging on health care expenditure and financing, with particular reference to the situation in Germany. Leidl's analysis challenges the popular expectation that population aging will be a major contributor to increased health care costs.

Instead, he argues that the complexity of the issue should push attention regarding resource allocation in the direction of flexibility within health care systems to accommodate these demographic changes.

The next four chapters deal with more specific issues at the level of macro-allocation of health care resources for the elderly. Mats Thorslund and Marti G. Parker explore various ways to meet the increasing demand for services by the elderly, including increasing efficiency in resource distribution and the establishment of public commissions to set health care priorities. In the end, they believe that the problem transcends such solutions because it is a matter of multiple sectors within both medical and social services. The priorities discussion therefore not only is urgent but must be widened to consider the interrelationships between sectors.

Ruud H. J. ter Meulen addresses how certain social processes, particularly the increased "medicalization" of old age, are threatening an important and fundamental value for health care systems: solidarity. As the aging process becomes increasingly subject to sophisticated medical technologies for acute care, solidarity between the young and old is strained through a diversion of resources away from the young as well as from long-term care. Ter Meulen argues that a two-tiered system of care—with a universally accessible tier of basic services financed by society and a privately financed tier—with an emphasis on care over cure will help limit medicalization of aging and maintain solidarity between groups.

The high-technology therapies that drive the medicalization of aging are the subject of Bryan Jennett's essay. He argues for the avoidance of simple modes of decision making regarding care for the elderly based on either the availability of high-tech therapies or on the patient's age alone. He discusses several factors that should be considered in decisions about medical treatments for the elderly and argues against age alone as a sufficient criterion.

Gebhard Allert et al. explore the meaning of old age as an approach to resource allocation on both the micro and macro levels. Looking specifically at the meaning of old age impeded by chronic disease, the authors examine the concept in relation to the life story—considered individually, within the network of personal relationships, and in the context of society. They argue that such considerations should be brought to bear on decisions regarding personal care as well as institutional health care arrangements for elderly with chronic diseases.

The next two chapters deal more specifically with issues regarding personal care for the elderly. Eva Topinková addresses family caregiving for the elderly, noting that families still provide the majority of care. Topinková traverses a wide range of considerations, including factors related to care recipients, care givers, and social changes. She concludes with implications for policy decisions centered on relieving the caregiving burdens on families.

Sarah-Vaughan Brakman narrows considerations of family caregiving even further by examining particularly the situation and obligations of adult daughters, who constitute the vast majority of family caregivers. Against a background of gender-specific roles within various cultural and religious traditions, Brakman analyzes the philosophical bases for filial obligations, arguing that gratitude rather than reciprocity should serve as the foundation for such obligations. From this position she draws out several implications for health care policy, particularly in favor of support for families trying to meet their filial obligations and for more gender equity in sharing the caregiving burdens.

The final two individual essays in this collection provide more specific illustrations of the tasks ahead for two vastly different kinds of societies—Hungary and the United States. Bela Blasszauer believes that only a good old age can make any medical efforts to extend life meaningful, or provide for harmony between generations. But Blasszauer paints a dark picture for the elderly in Hungary, noting problems ranging from inadequate institutional care to (not unrelated) high suicide rates for the elderly. Nevertheless, he believes there is room for optimism if social scientists and ethicists work together with physicians and policy makers to improve the elderly's quality of life.

W. Andrew Achenbaum provides a historical context to health care reform efforts in the United States. Achenbaum traces a history in which health reform measures occurred in fits and starts. Currently, reform efforts fail to take adequate account of the aging of the population and draw too sharp of a line between acute care and chronic disease. These issues must be dealt with adequately and publicly if Americans are not to squander what may be a last chance for meaningful health care reform for the foreseeable future.

Concluding this volume is a special report from the two-year research project "Care for the Elderly: Goals, Resources, Priorities." This report contains the recommendations of representatives from eight countries in Western and Central Europe and North America. The purpose of the report is to focus attention on the moral problems of care for the elderly in the coming years through six key recommendations. It is hoped that these recommendations will serve those making policy regarding future care for the elderly.

Mark J. Hanson

How We Care for the Elderly

It is said that the greatness of a nation is measured by how it treats its people. In many nations, the elderly are not given their due respect. But a survey of country reports from the Hastings Center–Maastricht Institute for Bioethics project on care for the elderly makes it clear that not only are the number of elderly growing rapidly but also the way countries care for them is an issue that none will any longer be able to take lightly.[1] The British report refers to a "demographic explosion," the German report describes "fundamental shifts" that will require new infrastructures for the elderly's care, and the American report foresees the future of care for the elderly as a "dangerous and delicate situation."

How have these problems come upon us? A review of the country reports reveals several quite interrelated factors as primarily responsible for increasing problems in care for the elderly: demographics, the structure of formal and informal health care systems and institutions, the elderly's largely negative social status, and developments in medical technology. Despite differences in the way countries configure those factors, there is much overlap in the way these factors affect the outlook for care of the elderly in each country.

Demographics

The demographics of the situation are unambiguous and virtually universal: the number of elderly and particularly of the oldest of old (over eighty-five) as a percentage of every reporting country's population is growing tremendously, and this trend will increase well into the next century. At present, the percentage of the population over sixty in the reporting European countries ranges from 16.6 percent in the Czech Republic to 23.1 percent in Sweden. Of these countries, Germany now projects the greatest growth in its elderly population in the coming century, with the percentage of citizens over sixty increasing from 20.4 percent in 1990 to 35.2 percent by 2030. By then, a full 6 percent of its population will also be over eighty. By 2040 most if not all reporting countries will have at least 30 percent of their population over the age of sixty. Sweden, being the "oldest" country, will likely not experience as great an increase in the number of elderly generally, but neither it nor the Czech Republic conforms to the otherwise near universal growth for the population over eighty-five. The growth in this age-group has been rising rapidly through this century, with greater increases expected. General trends indicate that the numbers of this segment of the population will be the fastest growing over the next thirty years, more than tripling in many countries.

Life expectancy also continues to grow as more children survive their youth and as medical technology finds new ways to prevent death—extending both living and dying. In general, life expectancy has increased at a greater rate for women than for men, although in countries affected by the Second World War, the degree of this difference may not remain as stark. The aging of the population may also be attributed to reduced rates of fertility, with Germany predicting an actual decline in total population in the early part of the next century if current birthrates continue. On the basis of these trends alone, health care resources everywhere will be increasingly strained, and countries will be forced to struggle with new ways to accommodate these developments.

The Elderly and Formal Health Care Systems

At this time, many health care systems around the world are undergoing reform to various degrees. Most European countries have some kind of compulsory, universal coverage and are now moving to accommodate private-sector institutions as well as other free-market mechanisms, at least in certain areas of health care. The Czech Republic and Hungary have the longest and most extensive experience with government-controlled health care, and they also have had the lowest percentage of their gross domestic products spent on it—6 percent and 4.14 percent respectively in 1992. The result for these countries, however, has been inadequate care for most people generally and a mixture of certain forms of high-tech medicine with poor overall conditions. Those European countries with greater financial resources for health care and somewhat more mixed financing systems have provided comprehensive care for at least most of the working population, but they are increasingly dissatisfied with inefficiency in their systems. The United States, in contrast, is recognizing the shortcomings of the free market for controlling health care costs, with 15 percent of its gross domestic product—a full one trillion dollars—now going toward health care. In all contexts, however, the imperative of reform is growing, with at least some attention being given to how nations are treating their elderly.

How is care for the elderly faring in this time of flux? In every country, the elderly are proportionately the heaviest users of outpatient and inpatient services. The Netherlands, for example, reports that 87.3 percent of people age sixty-five and older see a general practitioner over a twelve-month period, with an average of 6.7 contacts per year. Figures are similar or slightly lower for other countries reporting in this area. In Great Britain, where 75 percent of those over sixty-five visit a physician in one year, these visits account for 27 percent of the general practitioner's time.

In the hospitals, the elderly may account for up to a majority of all hospital admissions; for example, the Belgian report cites over 50 percent of admissions coming from those over sixty. The elderly also may occupy just under half of all beds (40 percent in Great Britain), and they generally account for about one-third of all hospital days (30.7 percent of days in the Czech Republic; 42 percent in the United States).

The report card on long-term care is mixed. Countries emerging from socialist systems, such as the Czech Republic and Hungary, have some kind of established structures of care for all ages. Unfortunately, the economies of these countries have been traumatized through their transition to a more mixed-market system; thus, quality of care for the elderly is poor and the distribution of resources uneven. The Hungarian report speaks of the elderly's "social isolation, loss of self-esteem, loneliness, depression, fatalism, and lack of dignity and prestige," with all this punctuated by high suicide rates in the older age-groups.

Wealthier Western countries may provide a higher quality of care for the elderly when it is available, but long-term care and other medical services for the chronically ill are often not adequately covered through the various delivery systems, and there are variations in quality as well. Generally, nursing home space is filled to capacity, with governments largely exerting pressure to minimalize institutional care of all kinds. The percentage of those over eighty in nursing homes varies somewhat across countries: 9.7 percent in Sweden, 11 percent in Belgium, 20 percent in Great Britain, and 30 percent in the Netherlands. Some of the variation in these figures may be explained by variation in types of long-term care available in each country. Sweden, which has a more extensive range of social services for the elderly, has various kinds of residential homes, sheltered homes, and group dwellings that are not included in their nursing home statistics. On the whole, however, every country experiences some kind of shortage of institutional space, with increased shortages expected.

In addition, Western countries have limited provision for government financing of long-term care. Germany, for example, provides four compulsory insurance systems as a "social net" for all of its citizens: general health care, accident, unemployment, and annuity insurance. But excluded from this net is coverage for chronic disease and long-term care. The provision for general health care, in other words, is oriented primarily toward the provision of acute-care treatment of persons with disease. The United States, which lacks general compulsory health care coverage, does have a Medicare program for those over sixty-five. But publicly sponsored long-term care (under the Medicaid program) is not available until all personal resources have been spent. And despite major efforts to reform the entire U.S. health care system, extra support for long-term care is not likely to be forthcoming. It is fair to say that in all countries, long-term care or coverage is either inadequate, unavailable, or requires (or will soon require, as in Holland) additional out-of-pocket payments.

The Elderly and Informal Care

The situation regarding long-term care, of course, puts added pressure on families to be the primary caregivers for the elderly. An estimate for the Czech Republic puts the percentage of dependent elderly cared for at home at 70 to 75 percent. Keeping the elderly at home and out of institutions is encouraged by pressures to keep health care costs down in light of shrinking budgets everywhere. In addition, this measure is sometimes supported by the moral argument that the elderly should be able to stay in their homes as long as possible. But because of the kinds of impairments the elderly are likely to suffer, care for them is labor-intensive and often requires support.

Home care, however, is becoming increasingly problematic for all countries—to varying extents but for several common reasons. First, economic and social changes have meant that women are more active in the workforce than ever before. This means that the number of families with an adult available to provide adequate day-to-day care for those elderly family members who need it is diminishing. Second, and not unrelated, the structure of the family is changing as well. There are many more single heads of households and fewer extended families.

Home care is not usually well supported by outside services, if there is any support at all. In the Czech Republic, only 4.8 percent of those sixty-five and older receive outside services; in the Netherlands, that figure is 10 percent, with Great Britain and Sweden at 7 and 8 percent respectively. Given the demographic projections and budgetary pressures, many countries are beginning to recognize that more creative solutions to care for the elderly must be found, including various kinds of nursing homes and assisted living arrangements, more support for ambulant care and services to assist families and other caregivers, and so on.

The Elderly's Social Status

That social support and institutional arrangements for care of the elderly are sorely inadequate is not fortuitous. This situation is derived in part from long-standing negative social perceptions of the elderly. There is a general equation of aging with frailty, weakness, and disease. Thus the elderly are easily taken to be a burden on the health care system and the rest of society generally. This is alluded to in reports from countries with socialist as well as capitalist histories but appears particularly prominent in former Communist countries. Of course, one might also appeal to deeper, more implicit explanations for inadequate attention to the elderly, such as humanity's general unwillingness to face reminders of fates that await those who grow old.

Despite this negative perception of the elderly, some manifestations of social attitudes reflect a more mixed view, and these vary with location. The report from Great Britain, for example, points to a shift in perceptions from the end of the 1980s—when the media portrayed the elderly according to a more negative stereotype—to the 1990s, which are seeing a more realistic and positive image. In the Netherlands as well, a benevolent attitude toward the elderly is noted. In many countries generally, the elderly are granted certain special privileges, such as discounts on transportation, utilities, and housing, as well as the protection of laws barring discrimination based on age. But these reports also imply an underlying ageism that is not readily amenable to broad-based policy solutions. For example, in spite of a positive view of the elderly, the Netherlands reports pressures to "give new generations a chance"; having an elderly person as the head of a business makes one look "conservative" or lacking in initiative. In sum, then, the elderly's social status in the Western countries would seem to be, as the U.S. report describes, "ambiguous and full of contradictions." Nevertheless, certain policies can promote more positive treatment of the elderly by younger generations.

That being the case, active participation by the elderly in organized political groups would seem to be central to promoting more favorable policies. But except in the United States, such participation has been limited. The reports from the Czech Republic and Hungary indicate that the elderly have little political influence. In the Western European countries, influence is growing but has been limited more to social and cultural activities, and to political activities on the local level. Belgium, for instance, indicates a real growth of municipal "elderly councils," and Sweden reports pensioners' councils in virtu-ally every municipality. These groups typically serve to advise and lobby on behalf of particular items in government budgets, support for home care and other intermediate forms of care, a better quality of residential care, more housing, beneficial retirement policies, and so on. But only in the United States are the elderly a significant force at the national level, now playing a major role in current health care reform policy debates.

Conclusion

It would be difficult for anyone reading these reports to be tremendously optimistic about broad political answers to the many problems involved in care for the elderly. Few countries are seeing any serious public discussion of these issues, although this is gradually changing. The policy measures taken in most countries to date may be more fairly characterized as adaptive tinkering rather than fundamental reform, and they have both positive and negative consequences for the elderly. Positively, these changes include flexible pensioning, programs to prepare people for retirement, special housing programs, and, in some countries, increased coverage by public insurance for the frail elderly. On the negative side, the elderly in some countries are facing budget caps, reduction of hospitalization, reduction in certain kinds of medical coverage, and additional copayments for treatments. But the reports seem to indicate that such measures will be inadequate for the long term; more substantial changes both institutionally and attitudinally may be required.

The Swedish report notes that steps to improve the efficiency of existing arrangements may already have reached their limits and that only more significant expenditures or more explicit priority setting will enable greater changes. It remarks that even if one assumes that care utilization and health status for various age-groups remain constant, with no great changes in medical technology, the need for all forms of care and service will increase 10 percent in the health care sector and 13 percent in the social-service sector between 1991 and 2000. At the same time, there are no plans in Sweden, or in most other countries, to increase expenditures for the elderly to meet that growing need.

How needs can be accommodated will probably vary rather significantly among countries. In Sweden, for example, reliance solely on charity organizations to provide necessary care is unacceptable. This attitude is congruent with many other European countries, where there is more of an emphasis on government-sponsored programs. But this stands in some tension with their current reluctance to increase spending for the elderly's care. In the United States there is more of an aversion to government involvement in health care provision of any kind. The outlook for the elderly here is thus equally uncertain. The American elderly may be now better off financially than their counterparts in other countries, but there is growing pessimism that the future will be as secure.

A few reports discuss or imply that the need to provide better services for the elderly will require more direct attention to priorities and the overall distribution of public resources. This is particularly problematic in the United States, where even the mention of anything like rationing is considered to be politically damaging. The European countries may have an easier time making the necessary large-scale budgetary adjustments. This is reflected in the reports themselves. A major recent reform in Sweden transferred responsibility essentially from the medical-care sector to the social-services sector for both economic and quality-of-care reasons. At the same time, the Swedish government has appointed a committee to develop priorities in the health care sector.[2] The Dutch government has likewise appointed a committee to develop criteria for health care services in ways that respond to the "greying" of the population and the increasing need for limits without discriminating against the elderly themselves.[3] The committee explicitly stated that age should not be a criterion for allocation of scarce medical resources.

It is possible, however, that rationing efforts may entail that the elderly receive fewer acute-care medical benefits in exchange for better chronic and long-term care services. Most countries deny any explicit rationing on the basis of age alone, although it is acknowledged as an "informal" practice. In the United States, there has even been an increase in procedures such as surgery for heart disease and kidney dialysis that were previously unavailable to the elderly. While this occurs to a lesser extent in the European countries, it is a trend that may only exacerbate current economic difficulties, even as it benefits individual elderly persons.

A related issue requiring further consideration involves the development and utilization of medical technology. Both the German and the Swedish reports suggest the significant role technology has played in contributing to the increased demand for, and costs of, health care. Medical technology is a blessing through its increasing ability to save people from premature death. Yet, as more people survive to an old age, the health care system confronts a growing demand for services. One irony of this development is that people survive diseases that would have previously killed them, only to be faced with an even worse dying process later in life. This is most evident, perhaps, in the increasing number of people who now die of cancer, Alzheimer's disease, and other forms of dementia—diseases that place additional demands not only on the health care system but also on social and familial support systems.

The final implication of these country reports on care for the elderly is that change is both necessary and difficult. It will require comprehensive and genuine discussions of the goals and priorities of both health care and society generally. The trick will be to accomplish beneficial reforms in a way that recognizes the need for priority setting and yet accomplishes it without further diminishing what some European reports referred to as "generational solidarity." Indeed, such solidarity must be strengthened if nations are to achieve true greatness through care for all of their people.

REFERENCES

1. This chapter is a summary of several country reports from the research project "Care for the Elderly: Goals, Resources, Priorities," conducted by The Hastings Center in cooperation with the Institute for Bioethics in Maastricht, Holland. The countries and authors are as follows: Belgium (Carine van Wanseele), the Czech Republic (Eva Topinková), Germany (Gebhard Allert et al.), Great Britain (Malcolm L. Johnson), Hungary (Bela Blasszauer), the Netherlands (Anneke van den Berg Jeths, Ruud H. J. ter Meulen, Rob Houtepen), Sweden (Mats Thorslund), and the United States (Daniel Callahan).

2. Statens offentliga utredningar, *Vårdens svåra val: Rapport från utredningen om priorteringar inom häso- och sjukvården* (Difficult choices in health care: Report concerning setting of priorities in medical care.) (Stockholm: Ministry of Social Affairs, 1993).

3. Government Committee on Choices in Health Care, *Choices in Health Care* (Rijswijk, Netherlands: Ministry of Welfare, Health, and Cultural Affairs, 1992).

Harry R. Moody

The Meaning of Old Age: Scenarios for the Future

Does old age have any meaning? Does the prolongation of life really amount to a benefit either for individuals or for society? Or on the contrary have recent gains in human life expectancy been instead a prolongation of decrepitude, frailty, and a meaningless existence? No topic seems less promising for productive public debate than a discussion about the "meaning of life." Talk about "meaning" is notoriously difficult and divisive. Yet without confronting questions about the meaning of old age, we risk impoverishing public discussion of choices that we all must face.

Over a decade ago Bernice Neugarten noted the trend toward an "age-irrelevant"society.[1] Her point was that there is less and less consensus about the values or appropriate goals for different stages of life, including the final stage. It is no longer possible to say what a "rational person" might prefer with respect to medical treatment to prolong life, especially if the conditions for survival are drastically different from conditions that earlier gave meaning and purpose to life. The trend toward an age-irrelevant society has important consequences for the allocation of resources in public policy: namely, it erodes any consensus about the legitimacy of age-based entitlements, such as pensions and health coverage.[2] Yet collective decision making, at least on a rational basis, is impossible unless we can articulate good reasons for allocating health care resources that take account of ostensible needs of the elderly, and the question of what counts as a legitimate "need" is precisely what is at stake in questions about the meaning of old age.

On the following table will be found four discrete alternatives or "scenarios" that define four different approaches to the meaning of old age. The table also indicates in broad terms the kinds of policy implications for resource allocation that follow from each of these different concepts of the last stage of life.

1. Prolongation of Morbidity

The first scenario comes from an unpleasant but inescapable question: how do we avoid creating huge numbers of "Struldbruggs," the people described

TABLE 1　Four Scenarios for an Aging Society

Scenario:	The Struldbruggs	Wonderful One-Horse Shay	Life Span Extension	Meaning and Aging
Prospects:	Prolongation of morbidity	Compression of morbidity	Genetic engineering	Recovery of life-world
Key idea:	Meaning = Quality of life	Meaning = Successful aging	Meaning = Progress	Meaning = Accepting limits
Origin:	Stoicism	Being = Doing, utilitarianism	Francis Bacon, Condorcet	Natural law, ecology
Current impact:	Right-to-die movement	Modernization of old age	Prolongevity, human genome	Social supports, hospice
Authors:	Derek Humphrey, *Final Exit*	Fries and Crapo, *Vitality and Aging*	Roy Walford, *Maximum Life Span*	Thomas Cole, *The Journey of Life*
Policy prescription:	Termination of treatment and assisted suicide; shift resources to those with favorable quality of life	Postpone morbidity to terminal drop; shift resources to health promotion and productive aging	Shift resources from sickness technologies to biomedical research aiming to delay or prevent senescence	End bio-medicalization of aging; set limits on health care spending; shift resources to psychosocial programs

in *Gulliver's Travels* as living in a condition of dementia with indefinite survival? Optimists believe that medical technology and changing health habits together will create a healthier adult population as we postpone sickness further into old age.[3]

What do the facts show? Recent data suggest that life expectancy among the aged *has* risen.[4] The result is longer periods of *both* health and sickness among different subgroups of elderly. Under a pessimistic assumption, the period of morbidity will grow longer. For example, even modest medical technology—for example, antibiotics for Alzheimer's patients—can permit survival to advanced ages for those with very poor quality of life. If the meaning of "good old age" is defined by the quality of life, then allocation policies should favor easing termination of treatment on the basis of quality. What are the implications here for allocation of scarce health resources? One implication might be to adopt a more permissive attitude toward all forms of self-determined death, including active euthanasia and assisted suicide.

Until recently right-to-die advocacy has been dominated by the rhetoric of individualism. But in the United States, as in Western Europe, concern about cost containment in health care has loomed larger, and right-to-die issues have become intertwined with resource allocation questions.

Cost containment might be guided by the quality-of-life standard in indirect ways. An example of such a policy shift would be a judicial determination that the "best interest" of a "reasonable person" whose intent is not otherwise known is presumed to be termination of treatment under conditions where quality of life dips below some threshold. There might be a rebuttable presumption *not* to treat—for example, to withhold Medicare reimbursement from—Alzheimer's patients certified as mentally incompetent or who are suffering from some other identifiable ailment. Many will respond that there is a dangerous slippery slope here once we accept the idea that quality of life is a valid factor for allocating scarce health care resources in the last stage of life. But the point here is that the "slope" is actually an implicit claim about the meaning of life in old age, where "meaning" is understood as quality of life.

2. Compression of Morbidity

According to most biologists, the maximum human life span is fixed at something like 120 years. We may not yet be able to surpass that limit, but our goal should be to eliminate the signs and symptoms of aging that appear before the maximum age. The proper aim of medicine and public policy, therefore, is to intervene, perhaps even slow down the rate of aging, so that more and more of us can remain healthy up to the very end of life. Sickness or morbidity would then be compressed into the last few years or months of life, as envisaged by the second scenario, compression of morbidity.[5]

This second scenario assumes a fixed limit to life. But within this limit, it aims for a "modernization of old age" implicit in slogans such as "successful aging"[6] or "productive aging."[7] Under this scenario, allocation policies would favor medical research and health promotion intended to delay morbidity and make old age into an extension of middle age.[8]

If we take compression of morbidity seriously as a policy prescription, then it would commit us to shift resources toward health promotion in order to make more of the elderly population healthier for a longer period of late life. More specifically, it would require us to identify those interventions of proven effectiveness that might bring about the largest number of quality-adjusted life years for the greatest number in the population. This policy goal can be formulated in terms of the maximum-benefit language of utilitarianism. But other ethical justifications are also possible. For example, a proponent of Norman Daniels's "natural life course" view might adopt this line of thought on grounds that a healthy old age is a condition we should prudentially choose for ourselves from behind the veil of ignorance.[9] For those uncomfortable with utilitarian language, this Rawlsian formulation amounts to arguing that to maximize successful aging and healthy aging is more just than to allocate resources to those who happen to be sickest regardless of age.

3. Prolongevity: Life Extension

The third scenario extends the idea of progress by challenging the "natural" limits presumed under the second scenario. If 120 years of life is good, why isn't 150 years better? Indeed, why not try to raise the maximum life span of the species?[10] Instead of "normal" aging, we begin on the contrary to think of aging as a "disease" to be conquered and cured.[11]

According to this third scenario, the entire human life course is open to revision by new knowledge of the biology of aging, especially the genetics of longevity.[12] According to this scenario scarce health care resources should not be expended on incremental gains in life expectancy or improving quality of life or even on enabling more people to live closer to a maximum upper bound. Instead, resources should be directed toward basic research into the aging process itself. For example, perhaps gene therapy will provide a breakthrough permitting us to raise maximum life span.[13] The ultimate goal is indefinite survival under favorable conditions of technological control. The meaning of aging as we have known it through human history would change radically. Aging would be progressively postponed and eventually eliminated, a goal that challenges our current agenda for biomedical research.[14]

The prolongevity scenario would urge shifting resources away from "sickness technologies" in favor of biomedical research to delay or prevent senescence itself. Obviously, it would be inadvisable, were it possible, to push up maximum life span without curing conditions like arthritis or dementia. Were we to enable people to live longer while still decrepit, we would be back to the nightmare scenario of the Struldbruggs envisioned by Swift.

The prolongevity scenario, as a strategy for research or clinical intervention, works along several lines simultaneously. In essence, it regards aging itself as a disease, rather than a biological limit to be accepted. In the first instance it seeks to raise maximum life span, something never yet accomplished in human beings; and in the second instance it has to delay or eliminate conditions we recognize as "normal" aging. Accomplishing both goals together would require an understanding of the biology of aging far beyond what we possess today. But such understanding may come in the future: for example, by investments in the human-genome project.

It remains, therefore, a valid question whether or not prolongevity should be pursued deliberately.[15] The current policy preferences of the U.S. National Institute on Aging are clear: the institute is *not* interested in supporting research explicitly designed to raise the maximum life span but, rather, in improving the quality of life in old age. The National Institute on Aging, however, also supports research on the basic biology of aging, and that same research could well lead inadvertently to technological means of raising maximum life span as well as (it is hoped) delaying debilitating conditions of senescence.

4. Recovery of the Life-World

The fourth scenario assumes that the meaning of old age is to be found in the finitude of human life as a condition to be voluntarily accepted through collective action, not individual choice. As a result of such collective decision, we opt for something less than the maximum life prolongation that technology could provide.[16] In effect, this strategy rejects the "biomedicalization of old age"[17] in favor of what Habermas calls the life-world. The fourth scenario seeks intentionally to recapture some of the virtues of the traditional idea of "stages of life."[18] More broadly, the fourth scenario evokes an ideal of vital involvement and concern by the elderly for the welfare of future generations.[19]

This fourth scenario can perhaps best be understood by analogy with the environmental movement. Following the line of environmental ethics, we might argue that longevity, like economic growth, can reasonably be restricted for reasons of solidarity or intergenerational justice. The common good and the needs of future generations are values that support limiting longevity in any one generation. An allocation policy for health care in old age should embody such values by favoring social programs such as hospice or home health care over high-tech medical interventions that provide only incremental gains for those who have already lived a long and full life.

The watchword for the fourth scenario is *not* the reflexive antitechnology outlook of latter-day Luddites but the sentiment conveyed in E. F. Schumacher's recommendation of "appropriate technology." Under this scenario allocation of resources would favor research and development for technologies defined as "appropriate" precisely insofar as they support values of the life-world. This scenario is perfectly compatible with decentralized, small-scale health care technologies that lend themselves to the home environment: for example, patient-regulated infusion for pain control. This strategy represents a "soft path" for distributing social and health services in an aging society, an allocation strategy quite different from the "hard path" based on centralized technology and hierarchical control.[20]

The fourth scenario is akin to the first insofar as both agree that imposing limits can give meaning to the last stage of life. But in contrast with the first scenario, an ecologically inspired sense of limits insists that meaning is *socially* constructed rather than an act of *individual* decision. The fourth scenario sees the meaning of old age as something sustained from generation to generation, a participation in shared living and dying, whereby we transcend the limits of individual life.

Discussion of the Four Scenarios

The four scenarios represent very different views about what future is possible or desirable for an aging society. The first scenario, prolongation of morbidity, is deeply pessimistic in its acknowledgment of the frailties of age. It heroically seeks to return decisions about death back to individual responsibility, urging us not merely to accept limits but to impose limits on ourselves and thus give meaning to our lives. The nobility of this ideal has not ceased to attract thoughtful people down through the ages, from the ancient Stoics to contemporary existentialists.[21]

By contrast, the compression-of-morbidity scenario is optimistic about old age. Its optimism arises from an acceptance of limits in the hope that within those limits, human existence can be made to flourish up to the end of life. Here the robust confidence of scientific humanism shines forth through the project of modernizing old age by investing it with a meaning that extends the worldly activity of midlife to the fullest.

The second scenario also reminds us that in order to escape fate and take control, we must begin far earlier than the last act of life, through health promotion.[22] But the second scenario achieves its goal only if it proves possible to postpone *every* disease or chronic condition until just before death. Like the Strategic Defense Initiative ("Star Wars"), this strategy assumes we can eliminate accidents. Yet the whole project can be defeated by chance, by the inability to achieve total control, since it is unlikely that all systems of the organism will wear out simultaneously.

The third scenario, life extension, confronts exactly the same problem. What if something goes wrong earlier in life—not in youth or middle age but, say, at age sixty or seventy? "Something going wrong" is another name for accidents, which are bound to kill in the end. Furthermore, if prolongevity were successful, it would pose other social problems. Longer lives mean greater diversity, which is another name for inequality. Life span extension would intensify all inequalities and give rise to envy on the part of those who have less, not only less time to live.

Serious equity problems also arise under the fourth scenario, recovery of the life-world. Individuals concerned about health promotion could still aim for compression of morbidity, while biomedical research might at any time open up unexpected possibilities for life span extension. Wealthier, better-educated groups would still have access to technologies for life span extension. The resulting inequalities of life expectancy would be difficult to control.

Is There a "Natural" Life Course?

Each of the four scenarios can be understood in part by its distinctive attitude toward "nature" and what is "natural," as well as related ideas such as "natural death" or the "natural life course." In defense of a Rawlsian account of allocation of resources according to age, Norman Daniels is the most explicit in his reliance on an assumption of the natural life course as a background factor taken for granted in ethical debate. But it is precisely such an assumption about the natural that is increasingly subject to question, both from findings in the biology of aging and from the spread of cultural norms that erode any consensus about a natural old age. Indeed, it is just such an idea of nature that is rejected, in different ways, by each of the four scenarios described here.

The first scenario, prolongation of morbidity, is itself the product of a quite "unnatural" intervention: the introduction of medical technologies that permit large numbers of frail and disabled people to survive far longer than they ever did when living according to "nature" throughout almost all of human history. This "unnatural" prolongation of debility is what gives rise to a demand that such an existence is "undignified" and that human freedom should aim at shaping an old age more in keeping with both dignity and natural life.

One of the earliest, and still one of the most powerful, philosophical claims on behalf of nature appeared in ancient Stoicism. The Stoic philosophy, in both its ethics and metaphysics, argued that the human good is possible only when man lives "according to nature." But Stoicism, like today's right-to-die movement, also insists upon human freedom and reason. Reason becomes our natural birthright, a capacity whereby we determine where the path toward fulfillment according to nature is to be found in any given instance. On this account, a mere indefinite prolongation of life would not be judged natural, while voluntary, self-willed death could well be judged natural. Rational suicide, in short, can well be the proper choice to make. The determination of where right action lies is not found by looking to an abstract natural life course. Instead, it is to be found in a quality-of-life standard.

The second scenario, compression of morbidity, more than any of the other three, takes for granted that there is a natural boundary to the duration of human life. The human body as an organic system, we are told, is bound to wear out in a fixed period of time. Nothing seems more natural. But is the natural life course then vindicated? No, because according to the compression-of-morbidity scenario a natural limit does *not* imply a natural life course as Daniels would invoke the idea to justify resource allocation. On the contrary, the whole idea of old age as a period of life appropriately demanding certain kinds of health care resources is an idea to be rejected. Instead, old age itself becomes transformed into a kind of prolongation of middle age.

What are the implications of this scenario for resource allocation? In the long run, as noted, the compression of morbidity demands shifting resources toward interventions intended to transform the meaning of old age as a stage of life. In the short run, it might seem reasonable to shift scarce health care resources away from frail or debilitated elderly in favor of others who would gain opportunities through health promotion and productive aging. But we shift the resources this way not because older people as an age-group have a lesser *right* to resources than the young but because the resources will do more good for others, not because of age-group competition but because we have transformed what is natural for old age in the first place.

Therefore, developed in this way, the second scenario by itself does not give us any basis for choosing among different stages of life because there is no natural life course to which we can appeal. Instead, the standard of good involved here is a commitment to refashion the last stage of life into something completely different from what a natural life course ever was historically. According to the compression-of-morbidity framework, the only thing deemed ineluctably natural is an upper limit on the life span itself. But the meaning of the last stage of life, and therefore the ethical basis for allocating resources among life stages, remains wholly unnatural and subject to human choice and technological intervention.

The third scenario, life extension, is the most explicit in its rejection of all ideas of nature that might determine ethical standards for allocating resources. There is perhaps implicit in an unconditional commitment to scientific progress a radical doubt about any fixed human nature at all. If we take this outlook seriously, there is no more reason to accept a natural life course than there is to accept "natural" sexuality or, for that matter, "natural" smallpox. The facts about nature or history are all susceptible to indefinite revision depending on human purposes. This is a Nietzschean scenario, filled with the intoxication and the grandeur of Zarathustra. There are no limits, including limits to life itself, to be taken for granted. The human good consists precisely in this capacity indefinitely to revise what we take to be good or a kind of life worth striving for.

If we are to *refuse* to develop technologies for life span extension, then our refusal will have to be a heroic one, not based on passive acceptance of limits but on a conscious decision, a will *not* to go down a certain path of technological development. The reasons for that choice will have to be made explicit. The reasons cannot be taken for granted or vindicated by appealing to the idea of a natural life course.

Finally, we come to the last scenario, the recovery of the life-world. Of all four scenarios, this embodies an image of the future most clearly inspired by a nostalgia for natural limits of all kinds. Old age, in traditional accounts, is invested with purpose and meaning, not only within the human life course but in the cosmic scheme. But with the waning of religious cosmologies, the metaphysical underpinning for this vision of the meaning of old age has disappeared.

In this vacuum of shared meaning, the recovery-of-the-life-world scenario is at bottom a story, a narrative that suggests how we ought to respond to technological advances that demand, or promise, a whole range of "modern" responses: individual control (scenario one), modernizing old age (scenario two), using technology to abolish limits (scenario three). The fourth scenario represents, in crucial respects, a rejection of the Grand Narrative of Modernity applied to the meaning of old age.

But after rejecting modernity, what do we find in its place? For all the reasons offered in criticism of the first three scenarios, we cannot now have recourse to a metaphysics of nature that would use natural limits as a way to vindicate shared meaning in old age. Does the deconstruction of natural stages of life then imply that the recovery of the life-world is, finally, nothing more than an illusion? Not necessarily. The deconstruction of nature is part of a wider "disenchantment of the world" (Weber). But it does not imply that narratives, grand or otherwise, are impossible; it only requires we choose them consciously and in dialogue with one another.

Conclusion

Under conditions of increased longevity and new medical technology, old age no longer carries a fixed meaning.[23] Instead, alternative meanings, such as quality of life, successful aging, indefinite survival, and collective acceptance of limits, each entail very different consequences for the allocation of scarce resources. This plurality of meanings will not be eliminated by appealing to a natural life course nor by Rawlsian arguments that separate the Right from the Good. On the contrary, public policy can and must take seriously a variety of different ideas about a good old age.

My purpose here has not been to argue for one scenario or another, nor to advance a single idea about the meaning of old age. Rather, it is to highlight the way in which different allocation choices presuppose very specific ideas about the meaning of the last stage of life. Certain ideas about meaning and value—for example, quality of life, successful aging, or intergenerational solidarity—are problematic because they involve difficult philosophical questions about the purpose of human life and especially the last stage of life. Both technocratic discourse and an exclusively procedural theory of justice try to evade these hard choices, but they will find that questions about the meaning of old age come back to haunt us in the end: the "return of the repressed," as Freud might have put it. Perhaps it is better to wrestle with these demons right now.

REFERENCES

1. Bernice Neugarten, *Age or Need? Public Policies for Older People* (Beverly Hills, Calif.: Sage, 1983).

2. Jürgen Habermas, *Legitimation Crisis* (Boston: Beacon Press, 1975).

3. J. F. Fries and L. Crapo, *Vitality and Aging: Implications of the Rectangular Curve* (San Francisco: W. H. Freeman, 1981); J. Fries, "Aging, Illness, and Health Policy: Implications of the Compression of Morbidity," *Perspectives in Biology and Medicine* 31, no. 3 (Spring 1988).

4. S. Olshansky, B. Carnes, and C. Cassel, "In Search of Methuselah: Estimating the Upper Limits to Longevity," *Science* 250 (1990): 634–40; M. Barinaga, "Mortality: Overturning Received Wisdom," *Science* 258 (1992): 398–99; G. Kolata, "New Views on Life Spans Alter Forecasts on Elderly," *New York Times,* 16 November 1992, A-1, A-15.

5. J. Avorn, "The Life and Death of Oliver Shay," in *Our Aging Society: Paradox and Promise,* ed. A. Pifer and L. Bronte (New York: Norton, 1986), pp. 283–97.

6. J. W. Rowe and R. I. Kahn, "Human Aging: Usual and Successful," *Science* 237 (1987): 143–49.

7. Robert N. Butler and H. P. Gleason, eds., *Productive Aging: Enhancing Vitality in Later Life* (New York: Springer, 1985).

8. J. F. Fries et al., "Reducing Health Care Costs by Reducing the Need and Demand for Medical Services," *New England Journal of Medicine* 329 (1993): 321–25.

9. Norman Daniels, *Am I My Parents' Keeper?* (New York: Oxford University Press, 1987).

10. Albert Rosenfeld, *Prolongevity* (New York: Knopf, 1976); G. J. Gruman, *A History of Ideas about the Prolongation of Life: The Evolution of Prolongevity Hypothesis to 1800* (Philadelphia: American Philosophical Society, 1966).

11. N. Shock et al., *Normal Human Aging: The Baltimore Longitudinal Study of Aging* (Washington: U.S. Government Printing Office, 1984); Arthur Caplan, "Is Aging a Disease?" in *Vitalizing Long Term Care,* ed. Stuart Spicker and Stanley Ingman (New York: Springer, 1983).

12. Caleb Finch, *Longevity, Senescence, and the Genome* (Chicago: University of Chicago Press, 1990).

13. W. French Anderson, "Human Gene Therapy," *Science* 256 (1992): 808–13.

14. Roy Walford, *Maximum Life Span* (New York: Norton, 1983); Michael Rose, *Evolutionary Biology of Aging* (New York: Oxford University Press, 1991).

15. Frederick Ludwig, ed., *Lifespan Extension: Consequences and Open Questions* (New York: Springer, 1991).

16. Daniel Callahan, *Setting Limits: Medical Goals in an Aging Society* (New York: Simon and Schuster, 1987).

17. C. L. Estes and E. A. Binney, "The Biomedicalization of Aging: Dangers and Dilemmas," *Gerontologist* 29, no. 5 (1989): 587–96.

18. Thomas Cole, *The Journey of Life: A Cultural History of Aging in America* (New York: Cambridge University Press, 1992); J. Burrows, *The Ages of Man* (New York: Oxford University Press, 1986).

19. Erik Erikson, Joan Erikson, and Helen Kivnick, *Vital Involvement in Old Age* (New York: W. W. Norton, 1986); John Kotre, *Outliving the Self: Generativity and the Interpretation of Lives* (Baltimore: John Hopkins Press, 1984).

20. Harry R. Moody, *Abundance of Life: Human Development Policies for an Aging Society* (New York: Columbia University Press, 1988).

21. C. G. Prado, *The Last Choice: Preemptive Suicide in Advanced Age* (New York: Greenwood Press, 1990).

22. F. F. Fries, L. W. Green, and S. Levine, "Health Promotion and the Compression of Morbidity," *Lancet* (March 1989): 481–83.

23. Peter Laslett, *The Emergence of the Third Age: A Fresh Map of Life* (Cambridge: Harvard University Press, 1991).

DANIEL CALLAHAN

Aging and the Life Cycle:
A Moral Norm?

Aging poses a peculiar puzzle for medicine.[1] As a biological reality, aging is an inherent part of organic life, affecting humans no less than animals, plants, and microorganisms. It is in that sense beyond the realm of medicine, a permanent backdrop to all of life. But aging is also ordinarily accompanied by disease, bodily decline, and disability. It is thus well within the realm of medicine, whose historical mission has been the cure of disease and the relief of pain, each much desired by those who grow old.

Yet is it necessarily true that aging as an inherent part of life is "beyond the realm of medicine"? If genetic engineering, or other scientific advances, could fundamentally change the phenomenon of aging—extending life significantly, for instance, to forestall the sicknesses of age—would it not then come within the traditional sphere of medicine? Why should medicine not attempt to manipulate the biology of aging rather than, as it now does, only the deadly and unpleasant clinical and psychological manifestations of that biological process? Should we go so far as to make the moral judgment that aging is in and of itself humanly unacceptable, a worthy candidate for scientific intervention, and even for eradication if we are clever enough?

There is, to be sure, a classical compromise response to these questions, first mentioned by the French philosopher Condorcet two hundred years ago and pursued most recently by Dr. James Fries: accept aging as a biological given but work medically to reduce the illness and disability associated with it. That heuristic ideal, the "compression of morbidity," seems the perfect answer; and it might be, in the best of all possible worlds. Unhappily, nature has not nicely played its assigned part, and so far, there is little evidence that any such thing is happening to any significant degree.

It has been little noted, moreover, that for the compression of morbidity to actually work, we would also have to forswear intensive medical intervention at the end of life. Yet might it not happen that many of those who lived so nicely and well until eighty-five would be unwilling to let go—just *because* they had lived so well—thereby setting the stage for a resumption of the now familiar technological battle against death? Another possibility presents itself also: if we do not achieve a compression of morbidity and lengthening life spans bring instead an increased burden of illness and disability, will we not then feel compelled to intervene more decisively in the biology of aging to combat that trend? Put another way, could it already be the case that we have come so far along the road in the extension of life, and so far along the road in the accumulation of the chronic and degenerative diseases of aging, that only some radical science can save us?

I want to suggest with these troubling questions just how difficult it will be to come up with good answers, but also just how portentous any set of answers is likely to be. At the least, with a growing proportion and number of elderly in every society, there is a critical policy issue at stake. To treat aging *as if* it is tantamount to a disease to be overcome is to open the way to an unlimited and insupportable claim on health care resources. If the diseases associated with aging bring about pain and suffering, as they do, then this is the basis for a time-honored claim to throw at them the same kind of research and resources as we throw at them at other stages of life. There are many who make exactly that claim, in the name of equality and age-blind social policy. If, in contrast, we want to pursue the idea of building policy on the basis of some kind of reasonable natural or cultural limits to such unlimited claims, we are open to the charge of ageism and to that of turning our back on medical advances that could improve the life of the elderly.

There is no easy way out of these dilemmas of policy, but it might help if we can sensibly frame the right questions to pursue about two principal ingredients of the dilemma: the nature of medicine as a practice and an institution, and of aging as a problem of biology and human meaning. Let me propose two broad questions we might begin with, each bearing on the other:

What understanding of the nature and goals of medicine is most likely to be helpful to the aging and aged in the future?

What understanding of the meaning of old age is most likely to foster the most helpful kind of medicine?

Of course what I mean to suggest by these two questions taken together is that there is, and must be, a reciprocal relationship between medicine and aging. On the one hand, the biological and technological possibilities of altering the aging process will shape our ideas and expectations about aging. On the other hand, what we want aging to be will help shape the research and clinical agendas of medicine. We cannot, in short, any longer think about human aging purely as an independent biological phenomenon (though on occasion it is worth trying to do just that). Human aging is, we now know, plastic to some as yet unknown degree and open to scientific change. We no less know that cultural attitudes and practices affecting our conceptions of the social and individual meaning of aging are open to change as well.

Aging is as good a place as any to observe the social consequences of medical progress, most notably the historical move from palliation to cure as a principal goal of medicine; and then from a narrow definition of health, focused on the body, to a broad definition, centering on the entire well-being of people; and from there to a static, nature-bound picture of the possibilities of living a life to a more open, wish-driven picture where nothing seems utterly impossible. What that process shows is not just medicine changing but, simultaneously, the culture with which it interacts. In the case of our culture, medicine is drawn to the promotion of autonomy and scientific innovation, the fashioning of an old age of one's choosing with whatever technology lies at hand, not bound by previous biological or historical models. The ideology of the anti-ageism campaign of recent decades is in part deeply rooted in individualism, celebrating the diversity and heterogeneity of the old—not what they share, the fact that they are at the end, not the beginning, of their lives.

The article by Harry R. Moody in this volume skillfully sets forth some different scenarios about the elderly and the allocation of resources, each of them drawing upon different notions of how we might think about aging and health care. I want to suggest another cut at the issues, complementing his but moving in a somewhat different direction. Two different models of the goals of medicine and the response to aging can be discerned, not formally articulated perhaps but nonetheless implicit in some familiar ways of discussing the problem. I will call one of these models progressive incrementalism and the other life cycle traditionalism.

Progressive Incrementalism

By the term "progressive incrementalism" I mean an approach to aging that is dedicated to unlimited progress in the long run but cultivates small, incremental steps in the short run. Average life expectancy can be increased to an unknown extent, but for the time being it is sufficient to add additional years slowly. And if a full compression of morbidity is not yet on the horizon, there is no reason we can't do something about osteoporosis, Alzheimer's disease, and arthritis in the reasonably near future. More generally, progressive incrementalism is sustained by the belief that medicine has no final inherent teleological goal for the elderly and that it can and ought to go as far as we want it to go. There are no intrinsic biological limits—or at least we will not know them unless we keep pushing the present limits, which always seem to give way—and there are no necessary moral limits, assuming we use ordinary common sense and sociomedical prudence along the way. There is no reason we should not seek both to extend average life expectancy indefinitely and to aim for a compression of morbidity along the way.

There is a social dimension to this incrementalism. It is, first of all, thought dangerous to think of the elderly in the aggregate as a discrete group or to think of individual elderly in general terms. Here the individualism of anti-ageism comes to the fore, arguing that for policy purposes age is no more relevant than height, eye color, or ethnicity. Just as medicine should have unlimited horizons in treating the elderly, so our culture should focus on the possibilities of individual development in the elderly, shorn of stereotypes or fixed boundaries. We need not worry about intergenerational strife because we will all pass through each stage of life: the sensible young will not see themselves in competition with the needy old but will see in the old their own future lives.

Progressive incrementalism, in short, combines a view of medicine and its possibilities with a view of aging and its possibilities. They work together, each stimulating the other: medical progress provokes new visions of what old age could be, and what people hope for from old age is an impetus to medicine to provide it.

Life Cycle Traditionalism

An alternative view I call life cycle traditionalism. It is traditional in that it does not entertain unlimited progress as a goal of medicine or a goal of aging. It is based on the biological rhythm of the life cycle as a way of providing a biological boundary to medical aspiration. This view looks to find a decent harmony between the present biological reality of the life cycle as an important characteristic of all living organisms—even if the length of that cycle varies— and the feasible, affordable goals of medicine. This view need not deny that considerable future progress in longevity is possible. What it does deny is that such progress will be of great human benefit, even if it may satisfy the wishes of some individuals. Neither does it deny the value of aiming for a compression of morbidity, even though it holds that there is nothing in nature, or the evidence to date, to suggest that compression will easily be obtained. It would, however, point out that if longevity and a compression of morbidity are sought simultaneously, the outcomes of the former may continually undermine the achievement of the latter.

The goals of medicine that lie behind life cycle traditionalism are to help people remain in good health within the boundaries of a finite life span and to help them cope well with the poor health they may have. It is thus a more modest view of medicine's appropriate goals, aiming to restore and maintain health rather than substantially improve the human condition. At the same time, it does not treat aging as a disaster to be overcome but a condition to be alleviated and ameliorated. Even though individual elderly people will differ in their physical and mental condition, they share the common trait of being elderly, that is, proportionately much closer to the end of their life cycle than to its beginning or middle; and as a consequence they are more subject to illness and death than younger people. Old age combines a biological stage in life and a social status in society, and it is not inappropriate that they be understood as intertwined. The same is true of every other age-group.

For policy purposes, the group characteristics of the elderly are as important as their individual variations. Those characteristics legitimate age-based entitlement and welfare programs as well as social policies designed to help the elderly maintain social respect. They could also be used to sanction a limit to those entitlements in the face of resource scarcity. The campaign against stereotyping the old as demented, frail, and burdensome is legitimate and needed. But there is a difference between a stereotype and a valid policy generalization. All elderly are not demented or frail. Yet it is a valid generalization to say that the elderly are a greater risk for dementia and frailty than young people—and thus to devise special policies to help the elderly, based on those generalizations.

Setting a Course for the Future

The two contrasting models I have offered differ both in their interpretation of the proper goal of medicine and in the meaning of old age. Progressive incrementalism has soaked up the optimism and ambition of modern science, its sense of wonder and hope in the face of a sometimes hostile nature. The nature that brings human beings down at the end of their lives can be changed. For its part, the meaning of old age is no less malleable, and medical progress can, together with enlightened social policy, change that meaning. Progressive incrementalism is of course the dominant ethos in scientific medicine more generally and not limited to the elderly. It implies an effort to overcome all biological barriers, from the beginning of life to its end; and it has no general goal, simply that of moving as far as is possible, wherever "far" might take us. Yet it is precisely this feature of progressive incrementalism that makes it so corrosive of meaning, so unable to offer a set of medical goals that will help make more sense of the place of aging in human life. It leaves that search for meaning up to individuals but manages nicely to simultaneously undercut that search by holding out a wide-open frontier of transformed aging, asking us, in effect, not to settle for aging as we know it—even while the aging we do know offers no radical transformation, only perhaps now a delay in the onset of the worst feature of growing old until a little later in the life cycle.

Life cycle traditionalism is skeptical of that pattern, noting in particular the difficulty that science is actually having in sundering the connection between getting old and getting sick, in overcoming the sheer stubbornness of those chronic and degenerative conditions that mark our modernized old age; and it sees no special reason to indulge the dream of a transformed old age. It notes as well a certain perversity about the progress we have actually witnessed: there has not been a heightened or rejuvenated appreciation of the social role of the elderly because of their longer lives and larger number. Instead, because of a pervasive ambivalence about whether old age is to be fought, rejected, and resisted, or graciously accepted and embraced, old age has been robbed of any substantive meaning it might have once had as an honored stage in an inevitable life cycle. Apart from ideological commitments, no one really knows now what to make of old age.

My own bias is that the life cycle perspective remains the most promising way of making medical and human sense of our aging. That perspective has three distinct assets. The first is that it remains the most compatible medically with the results to date of efforts to overcome the disabilities of old age, still more hope than reality. While much enthusiasm has been invested in the dream of a compression of morbidity prior to death, the evidence of movement in that direction is scanty indeed. So far, the longer life that is the fruit of the great gain in longevity over the past century has shown an increased, not decreased, burden of sickness and disability; those over eighty-five are particularly burdened (even if many do quite well). A life cycle perspective assumes, or should reasonably assume, that old age will see a physical decline prior to death and that up to 50 percent of those over eighty-five will likely suffer some degree of dementia. There is as yet no good reason to assume this general situation can soon, if ever, be overcome; and a life cycle perspective is useful in countering the endemic optimism of progressive incrementalism.

The second asset of life cycle incrementalism is that it offers a better framework than progressive incrementalism for individuals to come to terms with their aging, not holding out the expectation that the vigor of youth or healthy middle age will be indefinitely sustained—and thus not engaging in that most subtle but devastating disparagement of old age that the scientific fantasies inevitably feed, seeing it as nothing more than a condition to be overcome. While the campaign against ageism has been necessary and important, it has had, I believe, an untoward, unexpected consequence. By its stress on the individuality and heterogeneity of the elderly, it seems to have sought to make light of the fact that the old, however much they may differ from each other, are still old, that is, closer to the end of their life than to the beginning. Progressive incrementalism nurtures the ambition to pacify aging, to break the hold of the life cycle. An important, harmful consequence of the hope thus engendered is to create a profound uncertainty about whether aging is to be gracefully accepted or vigorously fought. Life cycle traditionalism pushes us toward acceptance; and acceptance makes the inevitability of aging more tolerable than that of a fight which must end in defeat.

The third asset of the life cycle perspective is that it enhances the possibility of devising an equitable health care policy—by recognizing the relevance of age as a pertinent social category, by resisting the notion that the diseases of aging are just one more biological accident to be conquered with better medicine, and by accepting the possibility that an excessive individualism in thinking about the elderly could run roughshod over the needs of the young. Progressive incrementalism, by contrast, has shown itself unwilling to see age as policy-relevant; it has altogether resisted that way of thinking about health policy and the equitable allocation of resources. But life cycle traditionalism accepts aging as a permanent human reality and sees no reason why that fact should not have a place in thinking about resource allocation. It helps set the stage for trying to discover the forms and amount of health care most appropriate at different stages of life, working from there to devise an equitable, age-relevant policy.

These three assets of the life cycle approach help us to better understand as well what appropriate goals medicine should have in caring for the elderly. The goal of medicine in the face of biological aging should be, above all, the targeting of those physical and mental conditions that tend to rob old age of human meaning and social significance. Medicine cannot create that meaning, which must come from individual reflection and social policy and practices. But it can enhance the background physical and mental conditions necessary to make that task a little easier. Yet it can only do so if it strenuously resists that most powerful of all medical temptations, that of seeing a direct and invariable correlation between medical progress and human happiness, of conflating the quest for meaning and the quest for health. They do not go hand in hand.

Yet, having expressed by own bias, I confess that I do not believe there is a decisive argument to be made for either the incrementalist or the traditionalist approach. The former appeals to our modern love of progress and open possibilities, while the latter can appeal to a sense of human finitude and a certain skepticism that the solution to aging as a human phenomenon of body and spirit lies in scientific advancement. This is a long-standing struggle, which would not have lasted so long were there not strength in both perspectives. Moreover, if it is reasonable to believe that there will always be a dialectical relationship between the medical possibilities of changing and manipulating the process of aging and our social ideals about old age, then there is little reason to expect that either will, or could, remain static: one or the other will change, thus shifting the equation over time.

Can there, then, be a long-term solution to the problem of human aging, or are we fated to have time-bound solutions, reflecting the medical knowledge of the scientific moment and the social ideals (and ideas) of the historical moment? Our solutions will have to be time-bound, but that does not mean we cannot have some permanent values that will help us better make sense of and manage the inevitable medical and social shifts that will occur. Three such values seem imperative and realizable. The first is that of intergenerational reciprocity, the mutual obligation of the young and old toward the welfare of each other. The second is that of the centrality of the problem of meaning to devising our ideals of old age, that of meaning as a value and a social aspiration. These two values—reciprocity and meaning—are long-standing and familiar, even if the subject of debate. The third value I would propose is less familiar: the value of moderate and modest and reasonably clear medical goals for the care of the elderly. The present situation, where there no longer seem to be such goals, at least at the research level, offers simply confusion and aimlessness, a progressive incrementalism that is going somewhere, but no one can say where. Life cycle traditionalism, for all of its problems, does offer a direction, one that is not beguiled by the promise that old age will just get better and better. That is something to hold on to.

REFERENCE

1. This paper is an expanded version of an article, "Aging and the Goals of Medicine," that appeared originally in the *Hastings Center Report* 24, no. 5 (1994): 39–41.

PAUL VAN TONGEREN

Life Extension and the Meaning of Life

In this essay I will present some philosophical reflections on the desire for life extension, a desire that most gerontological literature as well as public discussion—for example, on resource allocation—seem to take for granted. Although life extension generally is taken as a statistical concept, I will consider it transposed to individual experience.

I will ask whether people really desire to extend their life and why exactly we think they do. For this purpose I will first distinguish between different kinds of desire; second, I will reflect upon the concept of a natural life span; and third, I will consider our relation to death. In all three cases we will be forced to change the subject of our reflection: not the extension of life but the meaning of life is what demands our attention. But let me first make a few comments on the task of a philosophical ethics, or moral philosophy, and especially on what should not be expected from it.

Different Kinds of Questions

Especially in a multidisciplinary undertaking like this volume, it could be advisable to make some remarks on what one should and what one should not expect from moral philosophy. First, because there is an important difference between philosophy and the other disciplines, especially the empirical sciences; and second, because that places some important demands on their cooperation in a multidisciplinary project.

It is clear that it cannot be the task of moral philosophy to provide us with empirical information on the possibilities of life extension. But I think— in contrast with many people, even with some of my colleagues—that moral philosophy also cannot be expected just to answer questions like, Are we allowed, or even obliged, to extend life, and to what extent and under which conditions? or, How much of the GNP can be spent on care for the elderly? A philosophical ethics cannot just answer the questions in the way society asks them. Philosophy, rather, is an effort to raise problems where they did not arise before, to look behind the questions people are asking, and to try to diagnose what those questions and the way they are asked reveal about our present condition. What, for example, does it mean that we are inclined to talk about the case of the elderly as a set of problems to be solved?

It is told about T. S. Eliot that after he had given a lecture on an important moral issue, a student came to him and said, "That was very well said, Mr. Eliot, but what are we going to do about it now?" Eliot is said to have given as his answer: "You have asked the wrong question. There are two kinds of problems in life. One kind requires the question, What are we going to do about it? and the other calls forth different questions: What does it mean? How does one relate to it?"[1]

It seems important to me to distinguish for human praxis three kinds of questions. There are the scientific and technical questions about how things are and how we can do what we want to do. There are the philosophical questions, which ask what it really means that we want to do this or that. And both kinds of questions should be dealt with in their own way, so that they may contribute to the solution to the third kind of question, the (individual, political, or juridical) solution to the practical problems with which everyday life confronts us. Reaching a synthesis of these different approaches—that is, a synthesis of explanation and understanding—is a cultural task, the fulfillment of which requires multidisciplinary research. But this presupposes that the different disciplines can work in their own way, and so it demands that (moral) philosophy not itself be reduced to a "problem-solving activity."

One could suppose that the utilitarian calculus does enable the moral philosopher to answer in a definite way questions on what we are or are not allowed to do about the extension of life. Does not this calculus enable one to count the costs and benefits and to make up their sum total?

I will not discuss all the problems of this calculus and its utilitarian background. I admit that most, if not all, of the uncertainties it has to deal with can be taken away by statistics and more or less scientifically founded blueprints for the future. I even will not talk about the fact that such a calculus is always a bureaucratic affair, that utilitarian ethics is not only an impartial but also an outsider kind of ethics, and that it causes by that fact an unbridgeable distance between ethical solutions and moral experience.

Of more importance in our present framework is the question how I ever could determine the advantage or disadvantage of something like life extension. That is, how could I ever measure the quality of the effects of our life-extending efforts? That looks easier than it is. One could think that we can easily determine if and to what extent the expected consequences of those efforts are desirable or undesirable. But this would require that we knew our desires, that we understood their meaning, and that we were able to rate them at their true value. If these questions could ever be answered in a more or less definite way, then the utilitarian calculus could afterward become possible. But I think it clear that people cannot but try to understand and appraise their desires time and again. This means that there will never be a moment where the calculus can be made up in a more definite way.

There is another point that is of more specific interest for the present discussion. The utilitarian calculus presupposes the compatibility of the needs and desires to be calculated. But the desire for life extension might be a form of our fundamental desire for life itself: the desire that makes us attach to our lives. And this desire is of a totally different nature than all other desires. It is a desire we *are,* instead of a desire we *have.* This fundamental desire is the dynamic force of the living body in which it is incorporated, and in the human mind and its conscious reflection it is the desire for meaning, for what makes life (and its extension) meaningful. It is only on the basis of this fundamental desire that we can desire all sorts of other things. In other words, we can *have* all kinds of desires on the basis of this desire which we *are.* Let us call—with Bernard Williams—this fundamental desire a categorical desire, a desire that does not presuppose anything but, rather, is the presupposition of all other desires.[2] Such an incompatible desire cannot be discounted in a calculus. It should not be brought to a solution; it has to be interpreted and understood. If the desire for life extension is a form of this fundamental desire for life itself, how could a calculus determine its value?

Different Kinds of Desires

Let us develop a bit more this distinction between, on the one hand, the many desires and, on the other hand, this underlying desire for life itself or for the meaning of life. How are the two related, and what is the relevance of the distinction for the issue of life extension?

To live is to desire; and in our life we desire all kinds of things. But whatever may be the object of our desire, an affirmation of life itself is always included in every desire. To put it differently: while desiring all kinds of things, life desires or longs for itself.

The extension of life is as desirable as life itself. Any desire desires always also the continuation or the extension of the desired. As I asked my children if they would prefer their life to be longer than they expect it to be now, they made clear that they took that for granted. And not only we and our children but also former generations will have known this desire. I doubt whether it is true what Daniel Callahan wrote on this in his article "Aging and the Ends of Medicine."[3] He says that in former cultures aging was conceived of as something that should be accepted and as a time of preparation for death. In contrast, our time is said to consider aging as a disease to be fought and rejected. I doubt whether we are radically different in this respect. I think that the fundamental desire for the continuation of life is not new but that technological developments transformed this desire into a certain kind of desire for life extension, a desire that directs the research to the causes of aging and the possibilities of life extension, as it directs also the demands for life-extending treatments. It is remarkable that life extension—or the slowing down of the process of aging—is explicitly mentioned as a (or even the) object of scientific research from the beginning of modern science. René Descartes mentions it, as well as Francis Bacon, who is said to have died from the consequences of one of his experiments in this research project. Scientific and technological progress was probably conducive to the crumbling away of religious interpretations of this desire for the continuation of life.[4] The desire took the form of its most promising fulfillments. And today we find it even exploited in commercials in which kitchen appliances are recommended as instruments to extend our lives. The desire might have grown and certainly has changed its shape. But it was there all the time: every human being has this desire for life and for the continuation or extension of life.

This does not alter the fact that even this desire can wane and come to an end. Many elderly people in fact do not desire the extension of their lives but say that they would sooner not have their lives extended. My children, who took the desirability of a longer life for granted, started to doubt as I told them about the possible troubles of old age. And although they wanted their life as long as possible, it was quite evident for them that it should not last forever.

This is not contradictory to what I said before, namely, that to live is to desire and that life, while desiring, desires itself. That to live is to desire means that there is a point in life, that something is at stake. While we are not talking about this or that particular desire but about the basic desire for life itself, it is very difficult, if possible at all, to say *what* this point is or *what* it is all about. We call it the meaning of life, but we don't know what it is. But that there is something at stake implies that, in principle, this desire can be fulfilled, at least can be imagined as being fulfilled, or can appear definitely impossible to fulfill.

I will try to develop this a little bit more and to show its relevance for our topic: the moral evaluation of our desire for life extension, which seems to be presupposed as self-evident in our discussion of what we owe the elderly.

The Natural Life Span

Some authors refer to a theory of a "natural life span" to answer questions such as whether human life can be or even should be extended and, if so, to what extent, and thus to what extent the elderly have a legitimate claim for the allocation of social and health care resources. The reason for this is clear: if there exists something like a natural life span, then there also exists a natural death, that is, a natural moment of dying. If we could determine that moment, then we would have a criterion that could help us decide on the permissibility (and the bounds of the permissibility) of life-extending treatment, on the required research for such treatment, and on the legitimacy of care claims. Some authors even believe in the importance, for ethics, of medical and psychological research for such a natural life span. For example Arthur Caplan, in his article "The Unnaturalness of Aging," claims that it is important to find whether aging and dying are natural because, if they are not, we should combat them as we combat other diseases.[5] I will not elaborate on this position but say a few words on the way Callahan defines this natural life span and then make some comments on the normative meaning of this concept.[6]

According to Callahan, the natural life span is the time that is needed by someone to realize what he finds important in life. At first sight, this looks like a description that has a different meaning for different people and so does not have any specific meaning at all. But in his article "On Defining a 'Natural Death'" he specifies this description. A natural death is, according to Callahan, a death that comes at that point in a life span when (1) one's life work has been accomplished; (2) one's moral obligations to those for whom one has had responsibility have been discharged; (3) one's death will not seem to others an offense to sense or sensibility or tempt others to despair and rage at human existence; and (4) one's dying is not marked by unbearable and degrading pain.

This definition describes the situation and basis on which people *could* resign themselves to someone's (or their own) death being at hand: if there is not too much pain, if one finds comfort with others, and—most important—if the dying person knows that he is discharged from his duties (his responsibilities for others as well as his life work). With this last condition a clearly subjective and relative element enters the definition. What someone will recognize as his duties, responsibilities, and commitment will depend on his life expectancy, on how long he expects his life to be. And this expectation is relative not only to the character of the person but also to the development of the average life expectancy in society. And for that reason, this definition does not indicate whether someone is *right* in thinking himself discharged from his duties, nor does it show whether someone in such a situation would *have* to resign himself to his death. This is important because, or to the extent to which, the ethical interest in the so-called natural life span is motivated by the quest for a more or less objective criterion in nature.

To call the life span needed to realize one's life goals "natural" and to give this natural life span a normative meaning is questionable not only because it is always problematic to deduce norms from (natural) facts but also because one runs the risk of conceiving nature in an ahistoric way. Neither the life goals, and the time that is needed for their realization, nor the average or maximum life expectancy are unchangeably determined. Even natural facts are changeable. Not only natural evolution but also human acting, and thus cultural (e.g., scientific) developments, can and will influence our natural existence and our natural life span, as they have all the time. This cannot but mean that such a natural life span cannot be used as a criterion to answer the question whether life-extending treatment or scientific research for life-extending possibilities is permissible, or to what extent resources should be allocated to it. Nature as such can never supply an argument against interfering in nature.

This does not mean, however, that the question of the natural life span is meaningless. The question can be useful when it asks for the conditions under which people can experience their lives as successful and thus meaningful. But an answer to this question is by no means an answer to the question of a natural end of life, let alone an end in the sense of biological or physical time. It seems highly questionable to me whether such a theory of the meaning of life could ever be "translated" into categories of time, let alone of physical time. Before that, we would have to elaborate a philosophy of the different life stages, their respective possibilities for meaning, and the different ways in which these are temporal. After doing that, we might be able to ask for their possible unity. It is, however, not easy to conceive of this unity, and it is even more difficult to interpret it in terms of a certain duration. Paul Ricoeur interprets human life as "A Story in Search of a Narrator": life would realize its meaning and come to its "natural end" as soon as the story is complete, which implies that it is not only told but also read, heard, and understood.[7] But such an interpretation refers to a certain *way* of living, an *intensity* rather than an *extension* or duration of life.

The search for a natural life span led us again, and now for the third time (after this same question was also raised through our discussion of ethics and our distinction of different kinds of desires in the preceding sections), to the question of the meaning of life, the question of what life is all about. But as long as this question which arises again and again is not answered, how could we ever hope to say something significant about life extension? Why do we really desire life extension if we do not even know what life is all about? Should we not become suspicious?

Our Relation with Death

If we do become suspicious, we start to suspect that we possibly do not so much want to extend our lives as postpone our death. Could life extension be a flight from death? Could the same be true of the supposedly more modest desire for the reduction of morbidity? A retired colleague told me that he went to a doctor because of problems with his legs. After an examination his doctor concluded that it was a matter of wear and said, "Well, you should know that I cannot make you any younger!" To which my colleague replied that this wasn't what he came for; he just wanted to age some more. Could even the striving for the enhancement of our vitality in fact be an effort to free life from a view of death?

But, one could ask, what would be the problem with this? What is the danger of fleeing from death? I think it would be dangerous when—or, better, it *is* dangerous because—this flight is an illusion that ends in disillusion. It is futile to run away from death. Whoever tries to do so will be caught somewhere else. There is a famous Dutch poem by P. N. van Eyck, which goes back to a well-known story. The poem is entitled "The Gardener and the Death," and it describes the futility of this desire for a postponement of death. In my own translation, it reads:

A Persian Nobleman:

This morning my gardener came, trembling with fear,
into my house, and said: "Please my lord, hear!

While pruning the roses up there in the court
I saw suddenly behind me Death, my lord.

I, terrified—away I ran
but still could see his threatening hand.

Your horse is fast, my lord; with him I might
reach Ispahân before the night."

He fled away, and later—still before the dark—
I met Death while walking in my park.

"Why did you," I asked him, as he kept silent,
"frighten this morning so awful my servant?"

A smile was his answer, and then he said:
"Don't blame me, it really was not a threat;

I just was surprised to meet here the one
that I had to go for in Ispahân."

Gerontologists and doctors argue for the importance of "more life in years instead of more years to life"; this means that the quality of life is more important than the extension of life, which is only a postponement of death.[8] In line with a long tradition in philosophy, I would add that an important constituent of this quality of life resides in our relation with death. I will briefly mention some examples from the history of philosophy.

Some philosophers explicitly state that human life as such is only possible when it is *zum Tode,* "towards death," as Martin Heidegger says: life is only human to the extent that it bears death in mind, as its last possibility. It characterizes man that he has, almost from the beginning, a consciousness of death; his death is "something" that every human being has to perform all by himself. One can avoid all kinds of possibilities in life, just by always reaching for other possibilities; but one cannot avoid death. Here there are only two possibilities, according to Heidegger: either one takes this last possibility (up)on oneself and lives *eigentlich* (authentically), or one denies, misunderstands, or forgets about this possibility, and then one sinks into *Uneigentlichkeit* (inauthentic existence). Since human life is determined by finiteness and death, the meaning of life cannot but be the meaning of this finite and mortal life. The meaning of this life cannot be found in the negation of its essential characteristic. To be able to realize this meaning, life will have to be oriented toward this last possibility, it will have to conceive itself in that light.

Pessimistic philosophers, on the one hand, present death as the last judgment of nature and the definite proof of life's meaninglessness; on the other hand, they always make clear that their understanding of this—that is, their way of contemplating death—gives them a certain relief. They view death as the proof of the wrongness and meaninglessness of life: for everything that matters in life seems to end with death, every effort is definitely refuted by death as meaningless. Whoever might take comfort in thinking that the fruits of one's life will be handed down to following generations is mistaken insofar as he hopes to find a possibility of meaning in this way: the future generations will die like us, and there will not be a final success. Finally the earth will perish with all the kinds of life it contains. According to these pessimistic considerations, finiteness is in contradiction to the possibility of a meaning for life. The ultimate consequence is that death is itself the liberation from the continuing threat of death. Real pessimism knows that "being born is an inconvenience" (as the Rumanian-French author Cioran writes). I could also refer to the words with which Friedrich Nietzsche relates the legendary answer of Silenus, the companion of Dionysus, to King Midas. Asked what was the greatest good of man, Silenus replied, "What would be best for you is quite beyond your reach: not to have been born, not to *be*, to be *nothing*. But the second best is to die soon." But if life, which death makes meaningless, is still bearable for the pessimist, then it is through this craving meditation about death.

Epicurus, on the contrary, tried to show that death is not our business: as long as we are there, death is not, and as soon as death turns up, we do not exist any more. So never the two shall meet. Therefore there is no reason to fear this impossible encounter. Fear of death is based on a mistake, that is, on the mistaken opinion that life and death are connected somewhere, for example, that after dying we could still suffer the loss of our lives. But these Epicureans reach their liberating understanding only through their contemplation on death.

Probably all philosophies are in this respect tributary to the teaching of Socrates, as it is presented in Plato's *Phaedo*: to live is to learn to die. Stoic philosophy gave yet another interpretation of this teaching. It is with life just as with the agreeable things in life: we have to be conscious of their finiteness to prevent disappointment. While enjoying our dinner, we have to be aware that there will be an end. In the same way we have to live in a *praemeditatio mortis,* a premeditation of death. Since death can take away from us all those things to which we are attached, we should realize that the meaning of life cannot be in those objects of our attachments. I am referring to the Stoic doctrine of *adiaphoria,* indifference toward those things that are beyond our power. Whoever wants to realize the good life and to find the meaning of life will have to acquire this salutary indifference.

Conclusion

The all too briefly summarized attention paid to death by philosophy (and the same could be shown for religious traditions) should at least warn us not to run away from death. If we ask to what extent we are allowed to, or even should, extend life, we have to realize that we can hardly answer that question as long as we do not know what life is all about. Besides answering the question to what extent the available social and health care resources should be allocated to the care for the elderly, we should ensure that part of those resources will be invested in projects that stimulate the reflection on what life is all about. And discovering this demands that we recognize the finiteness of our lives, that we recognize our death. Instead of running away from death in our efforts for the extension of life, we should think of death in order to gain more depth.

For this reason I conclude with a reference to Nietzsche, who lets his character Zarathustra say: "Die at the right time. But how could someone ever die at the right time, who never lives at the right time?"[9] The central idea of his book on Zarathustra (and maybe even the central idea of all his works) is the eternal recurrence of the same. Not the endless extension of life but its eternal recurrence. The import of this idea is not to extend life but to intensify it. The first time this idea appears in Nietzsche's works, it has the form of a moral investigation:

> What if some day or night a demon were to steal after you into your loneliest loneliness and say to you, "This life, as you now live it and have lived it, you will have to live once more and innumerable times more; and there will be nothing new in it, but every pain and every joy and every thought and sign . . . must return to you—all in the same succession and sequence. . . ." Would you not throw yourself down and gnash your teeth and curse the demon who spoke thus? Or have you once experienced a tremendous moment when you would have answered him, "You are a god and never have I heard anything more divine!" If this thought were to gain possession of you, it would change you as you are, or perhaps crush you. The question in each and everything, "Do you want this once more and innumerable times more?" would lie upon your actions as the greatest weight. Or how well disposed would you have to become to yourself and to life to crave *nothing more fervently* than this ultimate eternal confirmation and seal?[10]

Instead of a moral judgment on the permissibility of life extension, I conclude with the proposal to use this thinking about life extension in a moral way. Let the debate about life extension stimulate us to ask this other question: what is life all about, that we could, or should, or even cannot but wish that it lasts longer?

REFERENCES

1. Thomas Cole, "History and Health: Progress and Paradox," in *Health and Aging: Perspectives and Prospects,* ed. J. J. F. Schroots et al. (Lisse, The Netherlands: Swets and Zietlinger, 1988), pp. 45–63.

2. Bernard Williams, *Problems of the Self: Philosophical Papers, 1956–1972* (New York: Cambridge University Press, 1973), pp. 82–100.

3. Daniel Callahan, "Aging and the Ends of Medicine," in *Annals of the New York Academy of Sciences* (New York: New York Academy of Sciences, 1988), 530:125–32.

4. Gerald J. Gruman, "Longevity," in *Dictionary of the History of Ideas,* ed. P. Wiener (New York: Charles Scribner's Sons, 1973), 3:89–93. See also Leon Kass, *Toward a More Natural Science: Biology and Human Affairs* (New York: Free Press, 1985), pp. 299–317.

5. Arthur Caplan, "The Unnaturalness of Aging," in *Concepts of Health and Disease: Interdisciplinary Perspectives,* ed. Arthur Caplan et al. (London: Addison-Wesley, 1981), pp. 725–37.

6. Callahan, "Aging and the Ends of Medicine," pp. 125–32. See also Daniel Callahan, "On Defining a 'Natural Death,'" *Hastings Center Report* 7, no. 3 (1977): 32–37.

7. Paul Ricoeur, "Life: A Story in Search of a Narrator," in *Facts and Values,* ed. M. C. Doeser and J. N. Kraay (Dordrecht: Nijhoff, 1986), pp. 121–32.

8. A. E. Hellegers, "Reflections on Health Care and Its Possible Future," *Kennedy Institute Quarterly Report* 5, no. 1 (1979): 1–6.

9. Friedrich Nietzsche, *Also Sprach Zarathustra,* in *Kritische Studienausgabe* (München/Berlin/New York, DTV/DeGruyter, 1980), 4:93 (my translation).

10. Ibid., p. 570.

Anneke van den Berg Jeths and Mats Thorslund

Will There Be a Scarcity of Resources?
The Future Demand for Care
by the Elderly

One of the major issues in the debate about the future of care is how to keep costs under control while meeting the growing demands for care. Addressing that, especially on an international scale, is far from easy. How are we to determine what the demands for care will most likely be? Even if it is not possible to estimate the future number of dependent elderly persons with any precision, it is hard to ignore the most probable scenario: a substantial increase in the number of the oldest old.

What factors—demographic, cultural, economic—will shape the future use of health care services, and how much reliance should policy makers place on long-term projections of population, health status, and need for services? What instruments are available to different societies and governments to control the cost of care? These are the sorts of questions we must try to answer in determining whether, and to what extent, we face a growing scarcity of resources as the elderly population grows.

Countries participating in the research project "Care for the Elderly: Goals, Resources, Priorities," conducted by The Hastings Center and the Institute for Bioethics in Maastricht, have totally different health care systems. The Western European welfare states (the United Kingdom, Germany, Sweden, Belgium, and the Netherlands) have a mixed system of government regulation and free-market elements, while the Eastern European countries (the Czech Republic and Hungary) are rebuilding their health care systems in the post-Communist era. And the United States is looking to reform its strongly market-oriented health care system. Despite substantial differences among the participating countries, we can identify various conceptual frameworks of factors that determine the use of health care services. But a single, generally accepted theory about the use of services is not available so far. This sets limitations on our ability to predict the future needs for health services. For this reason, projections of service utilization are often based only on demographics. These kinds of projections will be presented for the Netherlands and Sweden. The outcomes are discussed in terms of trends in utilization patterns and government policies.

Conceptual Frameworks for the Use of Health Services

There is a long tradition of research aimed at explaining the use of health care. In these studies a wide range of factors was found to influence service use on both the demand side and the supply side. The most important determinant of service utilization is health status, both as perceived by the individual and as revealed by diagnoses. On the demand side of service use, the central questions addressed by these studies are: what factors (apart from health status) influence the use of services, and why does one person with a health problem visit a professional caregiver while another person with the same health problem does not?

Different studies assess the importance of secondary variables differently. Depending on the approach taken by a particular study, the relevant factors pertain to any of four domains: the demographic (age, sex, socioeconomic status, income), the social-psychological (motivation, personality, medical knowledge, attitudes toward health, satisfaction with caregivers—the "health belief model"), the sociocultural (norms and values in one's own group, religion, nationality, and ethnicity), and the financial-economic area (health insurance system, out-of-pocket payments).[1]

Often factors from several areas are combined into one model, which may also include factors on the supply side of service use, such as ratios of health personnel to population or distance to service location. The aim is to explain as much variance in service utilization as possible.[2] Taking into account both health services and social services, it appears that the most important variables on the demand side of service use are age, sex, household composition, education, income, housing, social network, domestic skills, development of technologies to enable care recipients to live independently longer, and attitudes toward health and illness.[3] On the supply side, a great many factors must be taken into account in projecting the future supply of services, especially government policy (system of health insurance and health care delivery, capacity regulations) and characteristics of suppliers (productivity, efficacy, efficiency, medical-technological developments, cooperation and substitution among services).

An important hindrance in this field of research is the lack of theory about service use. Moreover, because originally they were designed for determining inequity in the accessibility of services (created by an inadequate system of health insurance), these models are not suited for causal analysis of service use.[4] Despite the lack of theory and persistent inequity in service use, efforts to explain service use are going on. But a new goal is added: models of service use are now being called on to serve as planning instruments for the care sector. The results can be characterized either as computer simulation models or as scenario studies.

The Netherlands has developed a rather strong tradition in both these methods.[5] Attempts have been made to apply these models in Sweden also.[6] The methods have in common the aim of providing better insight into future trends in the use of facilities than do projections based solely on demographic factors. Comparison of the outcomes of these different studies, however, is strongly hampered by the fact that they rely on different sets of variables and parameters.[7]

Apart from the technical problems of modeling, the demands placed on input data are high. Detailed information about service use is necessary, as well as quantitative data about past and future trends of the influencing factors. Even in countries with well-developed records of service use, the availability of projections for determinants of service use is limited. Often only population forecasts are available to policy makers. In the Netherlands, however, there are also projections of income and education levels of the elderly and of household composition for the whole population, as well as studies of the likely future health status of the population.[8]

Against this background, then, we can explore the kinds of demands a growing elderly population will place on health care resources.

Projected Demographic Demand for Services: The Netherlands

Like all Western European countries, the Netherlands faces a growing elderly population in the decades ahead. The absolute number of people age sixty-five and over will rise from 1.91 million in 1990 to 2.17 million in 2000, an increase of nearly 14 percent. The number of people eighty or older will rise to 505,000 in 2000 (from 427,000 in 1990), an increase of 18 percent. Table 1 gives the detailed figures by five-year age-groups.

The Netherlands has a relatively well-developed system of care for the elderly. Compared to other Western European countries, a high percentage of the elderly live in institutions—in 1990, 9.3 percent of the population age sixty-five and older. Although the number of beds in homes for the elderly decreased in the 1980s and the number of hospital beds declined from 4.45 per 1,000 inhabitants in 1983 to 3.82 in 1990, the number of beds in nursing homes increased from 47,600 to 51,700 between 1983 and 1990. Ninety percent of these beds are occupied by people sixty-five years or older. A relatively

TABLE 1   The Number of Elderly People on 1 January 1990 and 2000 by Age-Group, the Netherlands (× 1,000)

	Age				Total
Year	65–69	70–74	75–79	80+	65+
1990	629	468	381	427	1,905
2000	648	555	462	505	2,170

Source: Statistics Netherlands, Population Forecasts 1993 (medium variant).

small number of elderly are institutionalized in psychiatric hospitals and in different types of intramural settings for the mentally handicapped.

The most important traditional kinds of extramural care for the elderly are care provided by general practitioners, home nursing services, and home help; physiotherapy; and ambulatory services for mental-health care (like day treatment in psychogeriatric nursing homes). Programs of "intensive home care" have been launched in recent years, so that even patients requiring complicated and time-consuming care can stay at home if they wish. Home nursing services for the very old (eighty and over) have been intensified, but the total number of clients has been reduced. In home help there has been a slight increase in the number of clients in recent years; the amount of help per client has been kept on the same level. Table 2 gives an overview of service use in 1990 by people age sixty-five and older.

Several semiambulatory services have been developed in the last decades. Day treatment in hospitals, temporary beds in residential homes for elderly people living in the neighborhood, night care in nursing homes, and sheltered housing for psychogeriatric patients are some examples.

TABLE 2   The Use of Services by People Sixty-Five and Older in 1990, the Netherlands (Percentages of Total Age-Group)

	Age				Total
Service	65–69	70–74	75–79	80+	65+
Homes for elderly	0.4	1.5	5.2	23.4	6.7
Nursing homes	0.4	1.0	2.2	6.9	2.4
Home help	4.6[d]	4.6[d]	11.8	15.3	8.4
District nursing	5.0[a]	14.9[b]	14.9[b]	34.8	14.6[c]

[a]60–69.   [b]70–79.   [c]60+.   [d]65–74.

Sources: Statistics Netherlands, Statistics of Homes for the Elderly 1990; SIG (Information Centre for Health Care), Yearbook of Nursing homes 1990; Ministry of Welfare, Health, and Cultural Affairs, Financial Overview of Care, 1993.

TABLE 3 Demographic Projections of Increases in Demand for Services and Care by the Population Sixty-Five and Older (Absolute and in Percentages) in the Period 1990–2000, the Netherlands

Service (indicator)	Capacity 1990	Percentage Increase 1990–2000
Homes for elderly (residents)	129,300[a]	18.4
Nursing homes (beds)	45,000[b]	18.0
Hospital care (days × 1,000)	7,200	15.2
Home help (clients)	160,700	16.4
District nursing (patients)	306,500	17.3

[a]Total capacity in 1990: 134,700.
[b]Total capacity in 1990: 51,300.

Elderly people account for a comparatively high consumption of hospital care. Although people sixty-five and older compose only 13 percent of the total population, their share in the total number of hospital days was much higher at 44 percent. In 1990 the number of hospital days for the age-group sixty-five to seventy-four was 3.21 million and for the age-group seventy-five and older, 4.02 million.

Table 3 projects the effect of the growing number of elderly on the demand for services assuming constant use per person.

As table 3 shows, the growing number of the elderly has a substantial influence on the demand for services, with an average annual increase in the demand for these selected services of 1.5 to 2 percent.

Such demographic projections only make sense if all other influencing factors are held constant, which is unlikely to be the case. Scenario studies about health status show that the prevalence of diabetes mellitus and chronic nonspecific lung diseases will increase, while, for example, prevalence rates of stroke will diminish (due to improved treatment of high blood pressure). For other important diseases in old age, the prevalence rates are assumed to be constant because the determinants are unknown (e.g., dementia), effective prevention programs are lacking (e.g., arthrosis, cataract), or the balance of positive and negative influencing factors is unknown (e.g., hearing impairment, depression). Besides different kinds of changes in prevalence rates, the future disease pattern will be strongly affected by the greying of the population.[9]

Nor is disease prevalence the only factor complicating projections of future service use. Huijsman's simulation model, for example, shows that the demographic projection of the increase in demand for home help in 2000 can be limited by 25 percent, given the expected increase in income of the elderly (0.8 percent annually), a possible improvement of the social network (an increase of 10 percent in the number of social contacts), and a possible increase in private home help (an addition of 10 percent).[10] On the other hand, the growing share of elderly living alone and a probable reduction of informal care (due to declining birthrates and the increasing labor force participation of women) will cause an upward pressure on the demand for home help. These factors will most probably have a considerable influence on the use of social services but are likely of minor importance in the use of medical services.

In the Netherlands the trends in use rates over the past decade show that the supply of services did not keep up with the growing number of elderly. However, adaptations in the care system were able to compensate for this partly: the decrease in the number of beds in homes for the elderly was partly offset by the increasing age at admission, and the decrease in the number of hospital beds by a reduction of the average length of stay.[11] These trends are not likely to continue, however.

Government policy in the Netherlands is aimed at replacing institutional care with ambulatory care. Under current policy, only the capacity of psychogeriatric nursing homes is to be increased. At the same time, innovations in care for the elderly are going on, like experiments with "individual-care budgets," case managers, and new mixtures of housing and care. One of the ideas is to replace much of the capacity in homes for the elderly with apartment buildings affording a mixture of housing and care. This is possible since 60 percent of the elderly in these homes are not fully dependent; they only need some assistance. In this way government and caregivers are trying to keep the availability and quality of care at an acceptable level. But the growing number of the elderly makes it very unlikely that the increase in ambulatory care according to present policy can make up for the diminishing amount of institutional care.[12]

Recently government policy in the Netherlands has also adopted possible financial incentives to reduce the demand for care, for example, the introduction of out-of-pocket payments and limitations on the previously comprehensive health insurance coverage.

Projected Demographic Demand for Services: Sweden

The demographic trend for Sweden is somewhat different compared to the Netherlands and most industrialized countries. Currently Sweden is the world's "oldest" country, with 17.7 percent of the total population age sixty-five or over. The total number of persons in this age-group, however, will not

Table 4   The Number of Elderly People on 31 December 1990 and 2000 by Age-Group, Sweden (× 1,000)

Year	65–69	70–74	75–79	80–84	85+	Total 65+
1990	443	394	320	220	149	1,526
2000	375	357	333	244	204	1,514

Source: Statistics Sweden, *The Future Population of Sweden 1991* (medium variant).

change between 1990 and the year 2000. As can be seen in table 4, the age-groups sixty-five to seventy-four will actually decrease in number. On the other hand, the numbers of the very oldest in the population are continuing to rise, as they have done for some time.

Since age is the factor that demonstrates the strongest link with consumption of social services and health and medical services, the increase in the numbers of the very oldest will in all probability be accompanied by a growing burden on the various services for the elderly. On the other hand, the projections indicating a constant number of people sixty-five and older to the year 2000 will not increase the stress on the Swedish pension system.

As in other Scandinavian countries, the public system in Sweden for providing social services and medical care is extensive. The elderly receive care in a variety of institutions, such as nursing homes, geriatric wards, and old-age homes. Table 5 shows the proportion of people by age-group in different kinds of institutions as of 31 December 1991. The table also shows the high proportion of the elderly who received home help from municipalities during the year. Over the last decade, however, the total number of recipients has

TABLE 5   Use of Services by People Sixty-Five and Over in 1991, Sweden (Percentages of Total Age-Group)

Service	65–79	80+	65+
Somatic long-term care[a]	1.1	7.6	2.7
Old-age homes	0.5	7.4	2.2
Home help	8.7	40.1	16.5
Service houses	1.1	7.0	2.5

[a]Nursing homes and geriatric wards.
Sources: Federation of County Councils, 1992; Statistics Sweden, 1992.

TABLE 6 Demographic Projections of Increases in Demand for Services and Care by the Total Population in the Period 1991–2000, Sweden

Service	Capacity 1991	Percentage Increase 1991–2000
Somatic short-term care (beds)	32,000	9.7
Somatic long-term care (beds)	45,000	21.8
Psychiatric care (beds)	13,000	8.4
Old-age homes (beds)	34,000	21.5
Home help (clients)	286,000	11.4

Source: National Board of Health and Welfare, 1993.

dropped. This development is a consequence of attempts to trim back and rationalize services and to concentrate resources on certain groups of the population—in this case, the very oldest.

Elderly people in Sweden use hospital care at a high rate. In 1991, 62 percent of all bed days in short-term, acute care were used by people sixty-five and older, although elderly people constitute about 18 percent of the total population. The group seventy-five years and older (8 percent of the total population) accounted for 41 percent of the total number of bed days in somatic short-term care.[13]

As discussed above, it is possible to offer various projections about future needs of care for the total population in all ages. Table 6 gives an extrapolation of the consumption of services and care by the total population in all ages up to the year 2000, based on the consumption in 1991 and the demographic projections for Sweden.

If one assumes that health status and care utilization in various age-groups remain constant and that no great changes occur in medical treatment and technology, then one can expect that the need for the different forms of care and services included in table 6 will increase 8 to 22 percent by the year 2000.

The projected increases in long-term care, old-age homes, and home help are about equal with the projections for the Netherlands presented in table 3. The difference between the country predictions for different kinds of hospital care can most probably be explained by the different bases for the projections—in the case of Sweden the projections are based on the total population, including all age-groups, while the Dutch projections are restricted to the elderly. This methodological difference will, however, hardly have any impact on forecasting the services and care mainly directed to the elderly.

The biggest increases are expected in old-age homes and somatic long-term care (nursing homes and geriatric wards), where the number of beds must increase by 22 percent to keep up with the utilization rates of 1991. There are currently no plans in Sweden for such substantial increases in resources, either in long-term care or residential homes. Rather, discussions and plans have emphasized investment in primary care and home help services. If institutional care is not increased, there will have to be even greater investments in outpatient care and services.

It is hardly reasonable to believe that such increases could be attained through increased efficiency. This is partly due to the fact that the 1980s already saw a great deal of rationalization, but mainly because such a large portion of resources must be invested in physical care and supervision. Such care and supervision take time and are labor intensive, regardless of whether they are provided by public or private agencies, by the county or the municipality.

Allocating Future Resources

Given continuing academic controversies about the relationships among mortality, morbidity, and disability and about methods of prediction, how far should policy makers rely on long-term projections? Even if the demographic forecasts seem to be fairly reliable, it is not an easy task to define the need or demand for medical care and social services. Nor can we be sure that today's resources are being used as efficiently as possible. Similarly, we can't say that the quality of care provided today is the highest possible; indeed, it is not too hard to find inadequacies. And in any case, it can be questioned whether projections of future need should be based on today's utilization patterns.

What is obvious, however, is that predictable demographic changes will bring an increased demand for services and care for the elderly. Even though today's younger pensioners are in many ways healthier than those of yesterday, it is difficult to see any signs that the overall need for care of the elderly is decreasing in the Netherlands, Sweden, or other industrialized countries. In the short run, the increase in life expectancy among the very oldest will in all probability be accompanied by chronic illness and disability that will require medical care and social services—care and services that will demand more staff. Developments in medical technology, which have the potential to improve greatly the quality of life of the elderly, will also in all probability contribute to increased demand for care and services.

We may not be able to predict in detail just what services will be required in the year 2000 and beyond. But we do know the kinds of services that will be required to meet the needs of a predictable growing population of the elderly. We can begin today to determine what priority the meeting of these needs ought to have and to design appropriate policies for allocating our resources.

REFERENCES

1. Anneke Klaassen-van den Berg Jeths, *Care Services for the Elderly—Determinants of Use: Present Situation and Future Trends* (in Dutch) (Utrecht: State University, ISOR, 1989), pp. 39–167.

2. R. Andersen and J. Newman, "Societal and Individual Determinants of Medical Care Utilization in the United States," *Milbank Memorial Fund Quarterly* 51 (1973): 95–124.

3. Klaassen-van den Berg Jeths, *Care Services for the Elderly,* pp. 64–65.

4. D. Mechanic, "Correlates of Physician Utilization: Why Do Major Multivariate Studies of Physical Utilization Find Trivial Psychosocial and Organizational Effects?" *Journal of Health and Social Behavior* 20 (1979): 387–96.

5. Robbert Huijsman, *A Simulation Model for the Care for the Elderly* (in Dutch) (Zeist: Kerckebosch, 1990); Ans J. M. C. Vollering, *Care Services for the Elderly in the Netherlands: The PACKAGE Model* (Amsterdam: Tinbergen Institute, 1991); Social and Cultural Planning Office, *Use of Services Supplied by the Public Sector* (in Dutch) (Den Haag: VUGA, 1992).

6. Mats Thorslund, ed., *The Need for Care of Elderly Persons in the Year 2000: Researchers Look at the Future* (in Swedish) (Stockholm: National Board of Health and Welfare, 1993); Mårten Lagergren, "The ASIM-System: A Tool for Monitoring, Evaluation, and Planning of the Long-Term Care for Elderly and Disabled People" (Ph.D. diss., Karolinska Institutet, Stockholm, 1994).

7. Steering Committee on Future Health Scenarios, *The Elderly in 2005: Health and Care* (Boston: Kluwer Academic Publishers, 1994), pp. 156–58.

8. Dirk Ruwaard et al., "Forecasting the Number of Diabetic Patients in the Netherlands in 2005," *American Journal of Public Health* 83 (1993): 989–95; Steering Committee on Future Health Scenarios, *Chronic Diseases in the Year 2005,* vol. 2, *Scenarios on Chronic Non-specific Lung Diseases, 1990–2005* (Boston: Kluwer Academic Publishers, 1993); Dirk Ruwaard and Pieter G. N. Kramers, eds., *Public Health Status and Forecasts: The Health Status of the Dutch Population in the Period 1950–2010* (The Hague: Sdu, 1994).

9. Ruwaard and Kramers, *Public Health Status and Forecasts.*

10. Huijsman, *A Simulation Model,* p. 286.

11. Steering Committee, *The Elderly in 2005,* pp. 91–129.

12. Ibid., pp. 153–55.

13. Stefan Ackerby, *The Importance of Demographic Development in the Utilization of Health Care* (in Swedish) (Stockholm: Ministry of Social Affairs, 1993).

REINER LEIDL

Effects of Population Aging on Health Care Expenditure and Financing: Some Illustrations

In Europe the impact of population aging has become a popular threat to the health care systems. Recently, 2,700 European "opinion leaders" working in the health field were asked to identify the most significant problem contributing to the growth of health care expenditure. The survey reported population aging to be the number one issue.[1] Much of the popularity of this response may be related to the fact that it is hard to blame someone in the health field for this problem.[2] But in contrast to this broad agreement on the significance of the population aging issue in the health field, a number of economists continue to protest that demographic change has only played a minor role in the development of current health care expenditures, and some economists even dare to say that this also applies to future developments. So will demographic change ruin our health care systems or not? This paper intends to shed some light on the alternative positions and to provide material for further discussion.

The paper is organized as follows. It starts with a view of the demographic situation in the European Union (EU) between 1970 and 2050. Methods to assess demographic impacts are introduced next. Then impacts on the capacities of hospital care, on health care expenditure, and on financing are illustrated for one country. A summary discussing health policy and research needs concludes the paper.

The Starting Point: Population Aging

Population aging means that the age composition of a population changes in favor of the elderly. Two typical demographic developments that can lead to population aging and that are found in many societies of the industrialized world are decline in fertility and increase in life expectancy. For a more accurate description of the aging process, however, more factors would have to be considered, such as the time frames of fertility and life expectancy changes, the age-groups in which mortalities change, and the influence of migration. Population aging may occur in populations that are declining, stable, or even growing in size. Both the age structure of a population and its total size are relevant when we consider the impacts of aging on health care capacities and on financing.

One useful overall indicator that reflects the composition of the age-groups in a population is the "dependency ratio." This indicator relates the sector of the population that is not of working age to the one that is. The indicator used here is old-age dependency, defined as the number of people sixty-five years and older divided by the number of people between age sixteen and sixty-four. (For data availability, some illustrations are based on the range fifteen to sixty-four; this will only account for a marginal difference, especially in the development of this indicator over time.) An increase of this indicator is likely to be combined with growing utilization of health care in that population. In social-security systems that are funded from labor income on a pay-as-you-go basis, increasing old-age dependency means a rising financial burden on labor—other things, such as labor force participation rates, being equal. When we interpret this indicator, it has to be taken into account that some people between sixteen and sixty-four do not work at all, some work on a part-time basis, and some of those working do not continue until the official pension age; thus the indicator does not report the actual relationship of the working and nonworking populations.

During the last twenty years, old-age dependency has been rising in almost all twelve member states of the European Union of 1994. With the exception of the United Kingdom, the 2050 ratios of all member states have been predicted to exceed the 1990 figures by more than 50 percent, with most of them nearly doubling (table 1). In the first half of the coming century, a steep increase and the highest level of old-age dependency are expected for Germany; because of the availability of demographic scenarios, this refers to the population of former West Germany only. Throughout the European Union, the increase of old-age dependency is significant, and it cannot vanish by internal migration.

In the following sections, health care impacts of these demographic developments are illustrated with the example of Germany, the country expecting the most serious impact from aging on old-age dependency because it is combined with a declining population size. The demographic development described in the illustrations is based upon a scenario developed by the German Institute for Economic Research. In contrast to the data presented for comparison on the European level, this scenario provides age-group-specific data that are compatible with the data available on health care utilization. This allows the

TABLE 1   Old-Age Dependency in the European Union Member States—Absolute Figure and Indices for Population (65+/Population 15–64, 1990=100)

| | Absolute | Indices | | | | | | |
	1990	1990	2000	2010	2020	2030	2040	2050
Belgium	22.52	100	115	118	141	NA	NA	151
Denmark	23.03	100	98	107	139	NA	NA	171
France	21.10	100	114	117	147	NA	NA	178
Germany	22.38	100	114	140	156	NA	NA	186
GIER*	22.10	100	97	152	156	202	234	NA
Greece	18.87	100	122	136	145	NA	NA	182
Ireland	18.42	100	93	90	101	NA	NA	166
Italy	20.83	100	116	130	144	NA	NA	182
Luxembourg	18.30	100	113	115	182	NA	NA	174
Netherlands	18.52	100	108	118	155	NA	NA	203
Portugal	18.76	100	109	114	126	NA	NA	178
Spain	19.75	100	116	116	128	NA	NA	196
UK	24.03	100	101	103	117	NA	NA	125

Sources: German Association of Insurance Sciences 1994; German Institute for Economic Research 1990 (GIER), scenario A.
*Reference population age 16–64.

link required for impact analysis. From three scenarios originally available, the one featuring the highest increase in old-age dependency has been chosen for presentation. This "worst case" will serve as the reference point for discussion of the potential impact of population aging in this paper.

Assessing Demographic Impact

Demographic impacts in the health field are, by definition, a difficult issue to deal with. They extend over long periods of time—demographic forecasts sometimes look more than half a century into the future. Impact analysis requires a combination of three components characterized by tremendous uncertainty: the demographic development (for example, what the birthrate will be in the year 2020); health care (for example, to what extent minimal invasive therapy will substitute traditional inpatient care); and the general economy (for example, what the per-capita income will be). Accordingly, restrictive assumptions are often made in analyses in order to reduce this complexity.

There are several ways to investigate the impact of population aging on health care and on expenditures. Models that explain health care expenditure have been used in retrospective approaches. They estimate the contribution of independent variables, such as, among others, the share of the population over sixty-five, and employ either cross-section analysis across countries[3] or time-series analysis and pooled approaches.[4] These approaches have provided useful insight on the historical impact of demographic change on expenditure, an impact that generally was found to be small. The explanatory approach has not yet been used to identify the demographic impact on health care alone, for example, on the total volume of hospital days. It is not suited to consider long-term effects of future population aging. Other authors have tried to identify the impact of demography by embedding it in more complex economic models. Comparative static analysis has been used to assess the marginal impact of demography in behavioral microeconomic models,[5] and multiequation models and simulation have been used in macroeconomic behavioral approaches.[6] The theoretical basis, empirical relevance, and transferability of these complex models to other country and time contexts need to be further investigated.

The most common approach to assess demographic impacts is much simpler: the health care utilization or expenditure per age-group of today's population is multiplied by a future population structure. While it is often claimed that this describes the "pure" demographic effect, we all know that this is a fictitious exercise. Why should the incidence of lung cancer per age-group in, say, thirty years be the same as today? And if there were too many patients for available hospital capacities, would length of stay for the average inpatient remain the same while some patients would not receive hospital care at all? But methodologically, there are hardly alternatives to the simple approach. Even if we try hard, all the epidemiologic and economic developments cannot be predicted reliably over the relevant time frames. So when the impact of future population aging is considered, the simplest approach leaves us by no means with a predictive tool but at least with a reference point from which further discussions can start.

Simple multiplication of demography and current utilization figures is also the method used in this paper. A number of quantitative examples of impacts are discussed in an illustrative way. The illustrations are based on what-if reasoning—that is, scenario techniques—and do not employ any inferences. Methodological issues in demography are not raised. No trends other than demography are introduced in the impact scenarios. For pragmatic reasons, health care impacts are, furthermore, only investigated for hospital care. This excludes, among others, the highly relevant but loosely structured and documented field of nursing and home care. Comparative studies in Europe have indicated that the informal-care sector is by far the most relevant one in the care for the elderly in some countries.[7]

The Impact on Health Care

For someone considering the impact of an aging population on health care, a first intuitive approach might be as follows: the number of people in older age-groups is rising sharply; with increased age, the amount of health care needed rises sharply; consequently, health care needs will skyrocket. This reasoning, however, disregards the weighted impact of population aging. The multiplicative approach outlined above requires us to consider the number of people in the various age-groups over time as well as age-specific health care utilization. The elderly make up a relatively small share of the population (11.3 to 15.7 percent in the EU in 1990),[8] and a considerable amount of health care is rendered to those under sixty-five (table 2). The relative level of the latter is especially important because in some cases the absolute number of people under sixty-five will decline, and so will the respective health care needs.

Figure 1 uses the German Institute for Economic Research demographic scenario until 2040 to calculate the corresponding numbers of hospital days needed. The calculations are based upon the number of hospital days utilized by seven age-groups in the German local sick funds in 1989. These sick funds cover about half of the population, and the utilization figures have been assumed to be representative for the total population. Hospital utilization is differentiated in terms of the seventeen major groups of the International Classification of Diseases (ICD). Details on the data as well as on utilization indicators such as hospital admissions and length of stay by disease and by age-group are reported elsewhere.[9] For hospital days, the three highest-volume ICD groups for the population sixty-five and older are circulatory diseases, neoplasms, and accidents.

The link of the age-specific and disease-specific utilization data with the demographic scenarios provides figures for hospital days expected for the population structures in the years 2000–2040. Starting from the total level of

TABLE 2   Percentage Distribution of Population, Hospital Utilization, and Health Care Expenditure by Age, Germany 1990

	Population	Hospital Days	Health Care Expenditure
Population 65+	15.3	44.5	23.5
Population 0–64	84.7	55.5	76.5

Sources: German Institute for Economic Research 1990; Federal Ministry of Labor and Social Affairs 1991; Federal Association of the Local Sick Funds 1994 (own calculations).

% change

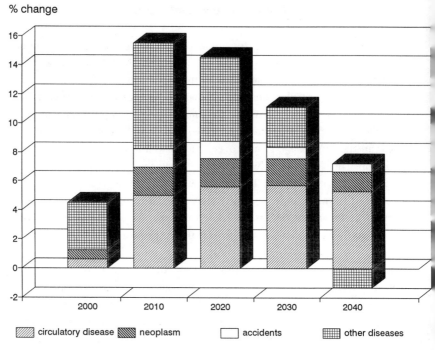

Figure 1 Demographically Induced Change of Hospital Days for the Three High-Volume ICD Groups, as Opposed to the 1989 Level, Germany (*Sources:* Federal Association of the Local Sick Funds; German Institute for Economic Research—own calculations.)

hospital days rendered in 1989 in Germany, fig. 1 reports the change in days expected for the three highest-volume ICD groups and for the residual group of all "other diseases." The rise in hospital days over half a century adds up to 6 percent; this includes the hospital days expected in the residual group. Considering that the norm for hospital occupancy in Germany currently lies at 85 percent, this challenge seems quite manageable. More relevant to policy makers seems to be the flexibility required by the hospital system in the medium term: in the ten years between 2000 and 2010, an 11 percent rise in hospital days would have to be dealt with. This is just the general capacity challenge. In addition, the disease spectrum is likely to change. A significant share of the medium-term growth is due to increases in the category "other diseases," which, as opposed to 1989, will decline to even a negative figure in 2040; this is due to the shrinking population under sixty-five. The two large health problems, neoplasms and circulatory diseases, feature a stable additional need from 2010 on. The issue of a changing patient structure in the hospital system is underlined by the fact that the demography of the hospital patients will change significantly, even more sharply than the general demography: 37

percent of the hospital days were rendered to patients sixty-five and older in 1990; using the above demographic scenario and hospital utilization rates, this figure increases to 57 percent by 2040. The hospitals will be full of elderly patients. In consequence of these trends, changes in the required service mix can also be expected.

A number of qualifications on the above observations must be mentioned. The use of stable utilization patterns is obviously not realistic for length of stay. Unlike any other indicator, length of stay has been linearly declining over the last thirty years. Extrapolating this trend will lead to negative length of stay by the year 2025. Thus, a nonlinear, long-term modeling of this indicator would be required in order to integrate its trend adequately. A further discussion of this issue is, however, beyond the scope of this paper. It has been shown elsewhere that the demographic impact on average length of stay—and on hospital admissions, the other component of hospital bed days—is small when compared with the time trends of these variables.[10] Second, the age-specific and disease-specific utilization patterns are likely to interact with the observed decline in overall length of stay; data on disease-specific variation of hospital utilization over time are still lacking. Another point is closely linked with utilization trends: the efficiency issue. U.S. authors observed that many elderly do not receive appropriate care;[11] this calls for an adaption of current patterns of care and thus of utilization rates. Furthermore, the extension of life expectancy has been taken into account in the development of the demographic scenario, but not with respect to utilization figures. It remains to be investigated how this dynamic factor will affect health care utilization. The problem cannot be solved by multiplying existing utilization with longer life expectancy; it has been shown that a significant share of lifetime medical care is required during the last year of life.[12] Accordingly, a more sophisticated extrapolation of utilization over the life cycle is necessary when we investigate the impact of increasing life expectancy.

Last but not least, it has to be remembered that this illustration refers to only one health care sector. Other care sectors, such as nursing home care, may be even more relevant to the elderly. On the other hand, there are also sectors that decline in relevance with increasing age, such as dental care. If declining utilization because of a smaller number of younger persons is not compensated for by increases in the intensity of care for this population, the additional health care burden caused by aging will be reduced.

The Impact on Health Care Expenditure and Financing

The illustrations of health care expenditures follow the same method used for hospital care. Because age-related expenditure data were not available over seven age-groups, only data for two groups could be used: expenditure for pensioners as an indicator for the population group sixty-five and above and expenditure for normal sick-fund members as an indicator for the population group below sixty-five. No disease-specific expenditure data were available at the total-population level. On the other hand, the expenditure of the two age-groups could be calculated based on data for all statutory sick funds, which represent about 90 percent of the total population. When looking at the impact of population aging, it again has to be considered that a large amount of current expenditure—about three quarters, even more than the share in total hospital days—is being spent on the population under sixty-five (table 2). The sick-fund data render a 1.7:1 relation between per capita expenditure for the older versus the younger group. In comparison with other countries, this is a quite small figure for this relation.[13] This low figure may be biased by the fact that the data used include expenditure for family members; dependents are automatically insured with the policyholder, and they may not belong to the policyholder's age-group.

The development of six main indicators is summarized for the period 1990–2040 in fig. 2. Changes can be directly compared by the index figures. Three demographic indicators are reported: old-age dependency, which more than doubles during the period investigated, and its two components, the population above sixty-five, which increases until 2030, and the working-age population, which declines continuously from the year 2000 on. Multiplication with 1990 expenditure figures renders the following picture: because of population shrinking—a 5.8 million increase in the elderly contrasts with a 16.7 million decline in the younger population by 2040—total health care expenditure declines from 2010 on, later even falling below the starting level. Per capita expenditure rises only by 9.1 percent until 2040, which corresponds to an average yearly growth of 0.17 percent—a differential impact that might be hard to identify in dynamic expenditure growth. Relating expenditure to the population aged sixteen to sixty-four renders a 31.2 percent growth over the fifty-year period. This corresponds to an annual growth of 0.54 percent, still a very modest increase. If the total increase in expenditure of about one-third translates into similar growth in premium rates in the German pay-as-you-go financing system, this would undoubtedly pose a serious political problem. Still, the increase occurs over a fifty-year period, where many other dynamics can be expected. A brief review of the last thirty years indicates that according to the OECD definition, nominal health care expenditure per capita of the population aged fifteen to sixty-four increased in Germany in the period 1960–1990 at an average annual rate of 8.65 percent; deflating this figure by the gross domestic product price index still leaves 4.50 percent.[14] The historical

index

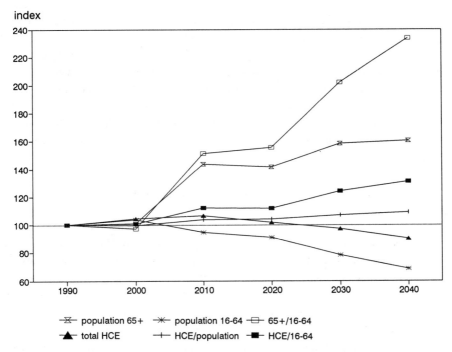

Figure 2 Development of Demographic and Health Care Expenditure (HCE) Indicators, Germany
(Indices, 1990=100) (*Sources:* Federal Ministry of Labor and Social Affairs; German Institute for Economic Research—own calculations).

expenditure trend by far exceeds the described future demographic impact. According to these data, population aging is not expected to be a major contributor to the growth of health care expenditure. In spite of that, financing problems will emerge when utilization and expenditure profiles remain constant in the long run.

It must be noted that the additional growth reported as an impact of population aging will also interact with any increase in the intensity of care or in expenditure that is caused by nondemographic factors, for example, by technological progress. The calculated additional growth of health care expenditure due to population aging then functions as a multiplying factor. Another remark concerns the distribution of health care expenditure among age-groups. In the scenario described, the share devoted to the elderly increases by a factor of about 1.8 until the year 2040. Future discussions on aging impact should thus consider age-specific distributional issues in the delivery and financing of care. Finally, it has to be remembered again that there are many qualifications to the above calculations. There were no budget constraints, no behavioral reactions, nor any trend other than demography in health care expenditure taken into account. An expansion of the health care technology provided for the elderly could significantly alter age-related expenditures. An increasing growth of the per capita health care expenditure for patients sixty-five and older, relative to the per capita expenditure of the remaining population, could quite appreciably affect expenditure growth indicators. Last but not least, general economic development has not been considered, and the growth of total labor income is a central determinant in any pay-as-you-go financing system.

Discussion and Conclusion

The investigation into the effects of population aging on health systems is a complex task. Starting with a brief review of methods to assess the demographic impact, this paper presented a number of quantitative examples concerning the impact on care, expenditure, and financing. In doing so, it referred just to one country, Germany, which faces the greatest aging challenge in the EU in terms of old-age dependency and a shrinking population. Impact descriptions were based on one—with respect to dependency, pessimistic—scenario. Impact was calculated by multiplying future population structures by current utilization and expenditure figures. No other trends were considered. Because of the illustrative orientation of this paper, no sensitivity analyses were conducted on the basic assumptions. Other limitations, imposed by the lack of factors—such as market mechanisms—that determine impact indicators, were mentioned. The assessment of demographic impacts has furthermore been constrained by the difficulty of predicting future developments on a sound theoretical basis and by the lack of data. Data requirements include sufficient differentiation of utilization and expenditure data by age, diagnosis, and type of health care sector, together with the availability of data over long time periods, in order to investigate historical trends and their determinants for the sound construction of future scenarios. Among other reasons, the lack of representative expenditure data for high-age patients impeded an analysis of the "double aging" effect: the growing proportion of elderly in the population and the increasing life expectancy of the elderly.

Yet, given all these restrictions, some results arose from the illustrations presented for the German context. A basic approach for the development of impact scenarios that account for demographic change and the major method-ological problems linked with this practice have been described. A number of quantitative results were achieved that at least qualitatively can be compared with other studies' findings on the impact of population aging. In addition, some of the results can be summarized for health policy purposes.

Other things being equal, the demographic challenge to hospital care in Germany described in the above scenarios can be characterized in terms of the task of managing, with significant medium-term flexibility, more appropriate care within the given capacities. Population aging is not expected to result in a need for more hospital capacity in the long run. The management of future hospital care must, however, pay attention to the significantly changing structures of the inpatient population with respect to age and disease. This may be linked with a growing intensity of care. Basically comparable results have been derived by a 1992 study of demographic impacts on United Kingdom hospital care for the period 1986–1995. The study, which employed age-specific utilization trends, found that demographic impacts vary widely across hospital specialties; it also underlined that demographic impact per se is a less important source of change than changing utilization rates.[15] Restructuring is more important than overall capacity planning in acute hospital care.

A remarkably low contribution of population aging to the growth of per capita health care expenditure has been described. An important assumption for this was the relatively small ratio of per capita expenditure for people above the age of sixty-five as compared with those below that age. The annual growth rate of per capita health care expenditure induced by aging is much smaller than the historically observed annual growth rates of per capita health care expenditure, either nominal or real. Though many qualifications and assumptions have been made in the illustrations, the result of a very modest contribution of demographic factors to the development of health care expenditure is fully in line with findings from other studies that employed different approaches and investigated different time and country contexts. The same result emerged from the explanatory approaches that retrospectively investigated this relationship for OECD countries in multivariate models,[16] and similar results have also been reported in a national study of Sweden, which employed the traditional multiplication approach.[17] Population aging, it can be concluded, has not been found to be a major cost-driving factor.

The relevance of the impact of aging increases when health care expenditure is not calculated per capita but related to the working-age population fifteen to sixty-four. The demographically induced growth in this indicator is highly relevant when financing aspects are considered. Other things—such as labor force participation—being equal, demography will contribute to financing problems in the pay-as-you-go system in Germany in the long run. The relevance of this finding is strongly emphasized by the fact that within the methodological framework used, the growth induced by population aging acts as a multiplying factor for all future increases in health care expenditure that are caused otherwise. Financing issues have been recognized as a priority issue in other studies, too.[18] Of course, aging-related financing problems of pay-as-you-go systems will be much more significant in the old-age pillar of the social-security system. It is sometimes argued that health care financing is a lesser problem in those systems where pensioners still pay premiums to health insurance funds, but this view only shifts the problem to old-age insurance. In any case, the political solution required for the financing of social security in old age is likely to codetermine policy on the financing of demographically increased health care expenditure. To design a health care financing concept that is stable in the long run, and not to contain demographically induced cost growth, is the key policy issue when we consider the financial impacts of population aging.

Population aging raises management and policy issues in both health care and its financing. But the scenarios illustrated do not support the simple popular expectations that population aging is a major cost-driving cause or a central dynamic threat to our care systems. Measures to deal with demographic impacts should emphasize the flexibility of the care system and the development of long-term financing concepts of social security in general. Neither the growing number of elderly nor their share in health care and its expenditures gives any reason to provoke discussions on discriminatory measures such as rationing by age. In the light of the need to control the nondemographic factors contributing to the growth of health care expenditure, considerations whether or not cost-containment measures disproportionately affect the elderly may, however, become a relevant issue in the future. This is in line with the priority need to develop concepts for more appropriate care for the elderly. Finally, further work is needed on the economic and ethical aspects of alternative designs to shape intergenerational equity in health care and other social-security financing, in order to tackle adequately the risks that population aging involves in pay-as-you-go financing systems.[19]

REFERENCES

1. Pieter Idenburg and Angelique van Vondelen, "Europese gezondheidszorg voorzichtig naar gereguleerde concurrentie" (European health care careful towards managed competition), *Ziekenhuis* 23, no. 13 (1993): 597–617.

2. Thomas E. Getzen, "Population Aging and the Growth of Health Expenditures," *Journal of Gerontology* 47, no. 3 (1992): S98–S104.

3. Martin Pfaff, "Differences in Health Care Spending across Countries: Statistical Evidence," *Journal of Health Politics, Policy, and Law* 15, no. 1 (1990): 1–67; Ulf G. Gerdtham et al., "An Econometric Analysis of Health Care Expenditure: A Cross-Section Study of the OECD Countries," *Journal of Health Economics* 11 (1992): 63–84.

4. Getzen, "Population Aging," p. S100.

5. E. Drissen and F. van Winden, "Social Security in a General Equilibrium Model with Endogenous Government Behavior," *Population Economics* 4, no. 2 (1991): 89–110.

6. Frank T. Denton, S. Neno Li, and Byron G. Spencer, "Health Care in the Economic-Demographic System: Macro-effects of Market Control, Government Intervention, and Population Change," *Southern Economic Journal* 55, no. 1 (1988): 37–56.

7. Anne Jamieson and Raymond Illsley, eds., *Contrasting European Policies for the Care of Older People* (Newcastle upon Tyne: Athenaeum Press, 1990).

8. Organization for Economic Cooperation and Development (OECD), Health Data File, version 1.5, Paris 1993.

9. Reiner Leidl, "Health Economic Issues Relevant to Countries with Aging Populations," *World Health Statistics Quarterly* 45, no. 1 (1992): 95–108.

10. Ibid., pp. 96–100.

11. Robert H. Brook et al., "Appropriateness of Acute Medical Care for the Elderly: An Analysis of the Literature," *Health Policy* 14, no. 3 (1990): 225–42.

12. N. McCall, "Utilization and Cost of Medicare Services by Beneficiaries in Their Last Year of Life," *Medical Care* 22, no. 4 (1984): 329–42.

13. Getzen, "Population Aging," p. S99.

14. My own calculations, based on data from the German Federal Office of Statistics and the OECD Health Data File 1993.

15. Alastair M. Gray and Nick Bosanquet, "Forecasting the Impact of Demographic Change: The Case of the British National Health Service," *Health Policy* 20, no. 3 (1992): 269–75.

16. Getzen, "Population Aging," p. S98; Pfaff, "Differences in Health Care Spending," p. 1; Gerdtham et al., "An Econometric Analysis," pp. 72–74.

17. Ulf G. Gerdtham, "The Impact of Aging on Health Care Expenditure in Sweden," *Health Policy* 24, no. 1 (1993): 1–8.

18. John R. Wolfe, *The Coming Health Crisis: Who Will Pay for the Aged in the 21st Century?* (Chicago: University of Chicago Press, 1993).

19. The author is grateful to Prof. Dr. J. A. M. Maarse, University of Limburg, for comments on earlier versions of this paper.

MATS THORSLUND AND MARTI G. PARKER

Caring for the Elderly:
Priorities for an Aging Population

In most industrialized countries, the needs and demands for medical care and social services for elderly people are increasing. There are several reasons for this. One factor these countries have in common is that the number and the proportion of elderly persons is increasing. This is especially true for persons over eighty years of age. The increase is expected to continue into the next century. Since it is the oldest groups that have the greatest need for care and services, this development is creating a challenge for welfare states.

Another factor is advances in technology that provide new possibilities for treating disease and alleviating symptoms and that can both extend life and improve the quality of life. Some experts contend that increased care costs are a result not so much of the increasing number of older people as of the increasing cost per capita.[1]

At the same time, many countries are experiencing a worsening economic situation in the public sector. This may lead to increased tensions between the different levels of the public sector—that is, national, regional, and local—as well as between different areas, such as medical care, social services, education, and so on. As administrators struggle to keep within their budgets, there will be more discussion on the limits of responsibility and the priorities for restricted resources.

What will this development entail? How great is the challenge? There are academic controversies about the relationships between mortality, morbidity, and disability and how to make prognoses of future needs.[2] Even if it is not possible to estimate the number of dependent elderly persons with any precision in the future, it is hard to ignore the most probable scenario—a substantial increase in the number of the oldest old and, with that, a substantial increase of needs for services and care in this sector of the population.

What strategies can be employed to cope with these growing needs?

Can Resources Be Used More Efficiently?

Resources can be rationalized through reorganization, through improving efficiency within organizations, and through better coordination between organizations. In many countries, the 1980s saw just such an improvement of efficiency. The changes made in Sweden have been described elsewhere.[3] Much of the slack in the system has, however, been drawn in. The central question now is, What gains can still be made? There is certainly potential for better quality, but it is doubtful whether further substantial savings are possible.

Can Technology Save the Day?

There is little hope that technology will radically change the health status of elderly people in the near future. We cannot expect any simple or inexpensive cures for cancer, arthritis, stroke, heart disease, or Alzheimer's, at least not in the coming decade. On the other hand, patients with these conditions often survive, but they need labor-intensive services.

Advances in technology have enabled us to perform some procedures more quickly, more safely, and with fewer resources. As a consequence, ambitions and expectations in medical care have been raised, and even very old persons are now receiving treatment that was not given previously.[4]

The potential of technology in home care, in the form of housing adaptations and assistive devices, is still not fully realized.[5] There is much room for development in this field, both to increase the autonomy of elderly persons and to improve the working conditions of the caregivers. Although much can be done to improve the quality of life—and some adaptations and devices may even be able to postpone the need for care services—it is unlikely that developments in this area will substantially decrease the amount of service needed. Limitations in the primary activities of daily living—eating, washing, dressing—demand personalized, hands-on service.

What Changes Can Be Made in the Social-Welfare System?

The 1990s to date can be characterized by the search for alternative ways to organize the care for elderly people, not only by making changes within the system but also by changing the entire system in several respects. "Throughout Europe, there has been a movement from unicentric welfare systems dominated by state provision to more mixed forms in which state provision is explicitly integrated and balanced with private and informal sources. This shift involves alterations in the dominant ideologies of welfare in which traditional social rationales are expanded to include economic and market criteria."[6]

The Swedish government wants to stimulate private initiatives and encourage competition, not only between private and public providers but also among the public providers themselves. Although intended to stimulate agencies to improve the quality of services, there are certain risks with increased competition, such as the duplication of services and a concentration on common problems, leaving the individual with unusual or complex needs without help. Certain costly services, such as rehabilitation, may be somewhat neglected by all providers.

The Swedish public is also being forced to raise their cost consciousness. The fees for services such as doctor's visits have been steadily increasing over the last decade. In other sectors, fees are now charged for services that were previously free. Means tests, rarely used in the past, are now used to set fees for home help and nursing home care.

These changes in the welfare system will lead to a more pluralistic system with more providers and with greater market orientation. Some people are concerned that these efforts to move public responsibilities (and expenses) to the private sector will not only increase inequities[7] but will also incur further costs that may offset the gains hoped for in recent reforms.[8] The changes will entail more paperwork and administration, the cost of which is partly responsible for the high cost of health care in the United States. Public providers have had the role of planning and managing services; many will now have to take on the roles of coordinating the different kinds of care and services[9] and of auditing and assessing service, both public and private. Procedures, standards, and quality assessment methods will have to be developed and implemented.

Are There Resources Not Being Utilized Today?

The increasing pressures on the system in Sweden have increased awareness of the essential role of informal care and the need to encourage and support caregiving relatives through financial incentives, social support, and respite care.[10] The governments of many European countries have moved quickly to encourage, mold, and incorporate family care into public policy.[11]

There is no doubt that savings can be made by utilizing informal caregivers. This development, however, may threaten the freedom of many women to hold gainful employment and, in general, their freedom to be active in society outside the home.

Younger elderly people represent an as yet largely unexploited resource. A volunteer organization has recently been created in Sweden that encourages younger pensioners to contribute to care in different capacities. Many countries, including Sweden, are discussing raising the retirement age.

Certain surveys have indicated that many Swedes would be prepared to pay more tax if they knew that the money was going to a better health care service. But at the same time, the political parties share a general consensus that taxes cannot be raised further. The possibility of allocating financial resources from other public sectors is very slim. All public sectors in Sweden are currently experiencing budget cuts. Any changes in reallocation would entail major changes in political goals and social policy.

The Total Cost of Services for Elderly People

Population aging is often referred to as one of the main explanations for the ever-growing demands on health care resources. Nonetheless, in most countries it is difficult to estimate the magnitude of this factor, since statistics are seldom broken down by age-groups.

In Sweden the total expenditures for health care as a percentage of the gross domestic product (GDP) rose continuously from 4.7 percent in 1960 to 9.4 percent in 1980. This was also a period of continuous growth in the number of elderly persons, especially in the number of the oldest old.[12] The period 1980–1990 showed a different pattern: a relative decline and a slower actual growth of expenditure in spite of the increasing numbers of elderly persons. In 1991, health expenditure was 8.4 percent of the Swedish GDP, which placed Sweden in an average position compared to other countries of the Organization for Economic Cooperation and Development (OECD).[13] The expenditure in the United States during this decade rose from 9.1 percent in 1980 to 13.4 percent in 1991. Even considering the methodological problems of measuring and comparing costs between countries, it is obvious that there have been some differences in the development in these countries.

There are several explanations for the slowdown of health care expenditures in relation to GDP in Sweden. The rationalization efforts of the 1980s may have contributed. Salaries for health care personnel were not allowed to increase at the same rate as other salaries during this time. Another factor is that several political decisions were made on both the central and the local levels about coordination and cooperation between different care providers.

Continuing this development of coordination, a decision was made by the Swedish parliament in 1992 to enact national reforms in the care of elderly persons. These reforms gave the municipalities full responsibility to provide

TABLE 1   Expenditure on Medical Care and Social Services (Percent of Gross Domestic Product, Sweden, 1992)

Medical care	(0–64 years)	3.5%
	(65+ years)	3.7%
Social services	(65+)	5.3%
	Total	12.5%

special housing for those people who require it. This meant that nursing homes, constituting about 70 percent of the total number of beds in somatic long-term care, were transferred from the medical-care sector (a responsibility of the county) to the social-service sector (a responsibility of the municipality). The social-service sector also had to assume responsibility, including financial responsibility, for other sectors of the former health care system, such as medical care for the nursing home residents. The main reason behind these reforms is that the previous division of responsibility between the health care and the social-service sector was not satisfactory either from an economic perspective or from the perspective of the quality of care.

In tables 1 and 2 we have tried to estimate the total costs for health care and other services for elderly persons after the reforms of 1992. Since there are no official statistics available yet, these figures should be seen as very rough estimates, based on various figures previously available. The statistics for the inpatient medical care are fairly reliable. The same cannot be said about the outpatient medical care, and can be said to an even lesser degree about the social services directed to elderly people.

As shown in table 1, the total cost for health care for all ages *and* social services for the elderly was about 12.5 percent of the GDP in 1992. The costs for health care for the elderly was about the same as the cost for the younger age-groups. Again, it should be remembered that in the 1992 figures, the costs for nursing homes (about 1.2 percent of GDP) are included in the social services (nonmedical care). The costs for all social services for the elderly were, then, about 5.3 percent of the GDP.

In table 2 the total costs for medical care (for all ages) and nonmedical care services for elderly persons are further divided between inpatient (institutional) and outpatient (community-based) services. Nonmedical care for elderly persons makes up about 42 percent of the total costs, rather evenly divided between institutions and community-based services. This means that nearly one-fifth of the total resources are spent on services such as home help, rent subsidies, meals-on-wheels, day care centers, and transportation services. About the same amount is spent on various institutions such as old-age homes, nursing homes, and group dwellings for people with dementia.

Health care costs for the younger age-groups were also about equally divided between inpatient and outpatient care. The health care expenditure for elderly persons, on the other hand, is dominated by inpatient/hospital care. Of all the services and care utilized by the elderly population, the social-service/nonmedical sector is the main provider.

In total, institution-based services account for about 62 percent of the total resources spent. From table 2 it can be seen that this imbalance between inpatient and outpatient care is due to inpatient medical care for elderly persons.

It is uncertain to what extent these figures can be generalized to other countries. Even if most industrialized countries share about the same demo-graphic developments, countries differ widely in the responsibilities of the public sector for providing health care and social services for elderly people. Another problem is the scarcity of statistics that differentiate between the various sectors and between age-groups, as presented in these tables. In most countries, the tradition of collecting and publishing statistics from the social-service sector is not as well developed as in the medical-care sector. Different countries also have different practices in the classification of costs, i.e., what is considered medical care and what is considered social service. The division between in- and outpatient services also varies between countries.

Nevertheless, we want to emphasize the importance of using table 2 (or an equivalent structure) in analyzing and discussing the developments made up to now and the potential for a more efficient and effective use of resources. Such a table is also useful in discussing future priorities both within and between the different sectors.

How Can Future Needs Be Met?

During the 1960s and 1970s, the number of recipients of home help and the number of beds in special housing and institutions increased at about the same rate as the number of oldest old in the population. But the 1980s called a halt in these developments. In spite of the ever-increasing number of oldest old, there was no increase in the number of home help recipients or number of beds in institutions. Instead, the emphasis was on efforts to improve coopera-tion and to increase productivity and efficiency. Of course, there is still room for improved efficiency. Since most of the slack in the system has now been drawn in, however, there is little hope for any further economic gains. Today those elderly persons who are admitted to institutions or who receive municipal

TABLE 2 The Proportion of Expenditure on Medical Care and Social Services by Age-Group and Type of Care

	Medical Care		Social Services	Total
Age-group	0–64	65+	65+	
Inpatient/Institutional	15	24	23	62
Outpatient/Community-based	13	6	19	38
Total	28	30	42	100

home help are really in a very dependent situation.[14] Consequently, if resources are not increased and the number of oldest old needing care does increase, the only solution will be either not to meet all these needs, or to transfer the responsibility to some other part of the public system, or to providers outside the public system, e.g., families, neighbors, voluntary organizations, or private providers.

Public Commissions Considering Criteria for Setting Priorities

Even if there are other possible "solutions" (e.g., further rationalizations or increasing allocations to care services), they will probably not prevent the necessity of making difficult decisions on the allocation of resources–difficult for both the caring professionals and the politicians. The method of setting priorities that was developed in Oregon[15] has definitely stimulated the international debate. The governments of Norway,[16] the Netherlands,[17] Sweden, and New Zealand[18] appointed committees with the task to discuss priorities in medical care.

Some of the criteria proposed in these committees include severity of disease, treatment effectiveness, and long-term benefits. These criteria are relevant and important, although not without controversy, in the field of acute, somatic medical care. There was also no assumption made that they should be relevant outside this area. Their usefulness, however, is limited for discussing social services or the relationships between service sectors.

Medical care is characterized, at least partly, by high technology and clear-cut goals. Outcomes are quantified in accepted measures (number of lives saved, years of life extension) or utilizations measures (number of reduced bed days for different groups). Social services directed to elderly persons, on the other hand, are characterized by low technology and diffuse goals. Outcomes are more qualitative and difficult to measure. The desired outcome is often that elusive measure—the quality of life. This does not mean, however, that we should refrain from studying these difficult areas; on the contrary, "given the vulnerability of this group, and the huge expense they represent, there is hardly any 'programme' in greater need of thorough investigation."[19]

The emphasis on the medical perspective in all of these committees presents a question: where does the responsibility of medical care begin and end? It is a difficult task to define the limits of the responsibility of medical care. In a discussion about the elderly population, the question is very pertinent. At what point does medical responsibility end and the responsibilities of the social services begin? There is no clear dividing line between aging and disease. To what extent are these criteria applicable to the main portion of the care for elderly persons, regardless of whether the care falls within or outside "medical responsibility"?

The general suggestions discussed by these committees have not yet been applied. If they were to be put into practice, what are the potential gains we could expect? And where, in which parts of the total sector of services and care, are the criteria that have been suggested for choices applicable?

The obvious overlapping between the health care sectors and the social services regarding the care of the elderly emphasizes the need for dealing with a wider perspective. If the medical-care sector tries to safeguard their restricted resources by defining the responsibility of medical care to exclude care services devoted to elderly persons, this will have repercussions on the social services as well as on elderly persons and their families.

The criteria proposed by these committees—for example, severity of disease and treatment effectiveness—are not applicable within other sectors, nor do they seem to be relevant for making decisions about allocating resources between sectors.

The Total Picture

If we, then, look at the total medical and social services for elderly persons in the different cells of table 2, we must ask ourselves about the interrelationships between the sectors. What happens when changes are made in one section or when resources or demands are transferred between sectors? How does this affect the total picture?

Through rationalization efforts and improvements in technology, lessons have been learned within certain sectors. As stated above, this holds true, for example, for acute somatic care, the community-based services, and the different kinds of housing for elderly persons. It is obvious that few of these lessons can be applied and generalized in other areas. The same holds true for discussion about priorities. It is essential that discussions of priorities—in the allocation of resources and the further rationalization of resources—are based on the different prerequisites in the different sectors.

As the various sectors of care begin to define and limit their areas of responsibilities, there is a risk that certain areas will be left out. Rehabilitation is one of these areas that falls between the scopes of medical care and social services. At the present time in Sweden, the responsibility for rehabilitation is divided diffusely among all the cells of table 2. The goals of rehabilitation are often neither curing or caring; rather, rehabilitation aims at improving mobility, slowing the disease process, and restoring autonomy to the individual. Rehabilitation is often labor intensive and thereby expensive, and the benefits of rehabilitation, like those of social services, are difficult to measure, in particular for elderly persons. Often we are dealing with symptoms that will intensify with time; rehabilitation only tries to slow down the inevitable deterioration. It is more difficult to measure the life added to years than to measure the years added to life. Nevertheless, it is essential that we continue efforts to clarify goals and assess progress in this area.

The care of demented persons is another example of an area that does not fall easily within the medical model, nor is it solely confined to social services. Medical competence is particularly needed in the diagnostic phase.

Conclusions—Expanding the Priorities Discussion

On the one hand, there is a need for the different sectors to discuss rationalizations and priorities based on the goals, prerequisites, and conditions within each sector. On the other hand, there must be discussions with a more global perspective that consider all of the available resources and that are based on all of the needs of elderly individuals. How can discussion be extended beyond the narrow confines of the directives that have been given to the national committees? How can the perspective be widened to include the interrelationships between sectors? How can discussion be stimulated in the social services?

The difficulty and complexity of discussing this wider perspective is intimidating and may explain the scarcity of open discussions up to now. There are no simple answers. A problem this complex cannot have simple solutions. We cannot expect solutions from a single discipline.

Until some years ago, there were no open discussions about priorities. Of course, decisions have always been made on the basis of certain priorities, either unconsciously or behind closed doors. The current economic situation, together with the aging population, has elicited a more open discussion. Today there are officially appointed committees in several countries.

In our opinion, there is a clear limitation if the necessary discussions are dominated by the restricted, mainly medically oriented perspective—first, because the criteria relevant to somatic medicine cannot be generalized to the nonmedical sectors, and second, at least in Sweden, because the discussion is applicable to less than half of the total care and services for the elderly population.

The current discussion of priorities in medical care has come to the fore in part because of the growing elderly population; therefore it is important that it is the needs of the elderly population that are considered in further discussion. The criteria that have been discussed in the national committees are complex and controversial in themselves and are not sufficient in the broader perspective of care for the elderly population.

REFERENCES

1. Robert G. Evans, "Reflections on the Revolution in Sweden," in *International Review of the Swedish Health Care System,* ed. A. J. Culyer (Stockholm: SNS, 1991), pp. 118–157; R. Leidl, "Health Economic Issues Relevant to Countries with Aging Populations," *World Health Statistics Quarterly* 45 (1992): 95–108.

2. Kenneth G. Manton, "Mortality and Morbidity," in *Handbook of Aging and the Social Sciences,* ed. R. H. Binstock and Linda K. George (San Diego: Academic Press), pp. 64–90; R. A. Easterlin, "The Economic Impact of Prospective Population Changes in Advanced Industrial Countries: An Historical Perspective," *Journals of Gerontology: Social Sciences* 46 (1991): S299–S309; J. Fries, "The Compression of Morbidity: Near or Far?" *Milbank Memorial Fund Quarterly* 67, no. 2 (1989): 208–32; Jack M. Guralnik, "Prospects for the Compression of Morbidity," *Journal of Aging and Health* 3 (1991): 138–54.

3. Mats Thorslund, "The Increasing Number of Very Old People Will Change the Swedish Model of the Welfare State," *Social Sciences and Medicine* 32 (1991): 455–64; Mats Thorslund, "Home Care in Sweden: Past and Future Trends," in *Better Care for Dependent People Living at Home: Meeting the New Agenda in Services for the Elderly,* ed. Adelbert Evers and G. H. van der Zanden (Bunnik: Netherlands Institute of Gerontology, 1993), pp. 96–114; Mats Thorslund and Marti G. Parker, "Care of the Elderly in the Changing Swedish Welfare State," in *Community Care: New Agendas and Challenges from the UK and Overseas,* ed. D. Challis and B. Davis (Aldershot: Ashgate, 1994), pp. 249–63.

4. Ove Lundvall, "Sjukvårdskonsumtion och Sjukdomspanorama vid en Medicinklinik Perioden 1953–1986" (Medical care consumption and disease panorama from a medical ward, 1953–1986), *Läkartidningen* 85 (1988): 4280–87; Ulf Gerdtham and Bengt Jönsson, "Health Care Expenditure in Sweden: An International Comparison," *Health Policy* 19 (1991): 211–28.

5. Marti G. Parker and Mats Thorslund, "The Provision of Assistive Technology for the Elderly in Sweden," *Technology and Disability* 2, no. 2 (1993): 45–49.

6. John Baldock and Adelbert Evers, "Innovations and Care of the Elderly: The Front Line of Change for Social Welfare Services," *Ageing International,* June 1991, 8–21.

7. Thorslund, "The Increasing Number."

8. Johan Calltorp, "Prioritering och Beslutsprocess i Sjukvårdsfrågor: Några Drag i de Senaste Decenniernas Sjukvårdspolitik" (Priority setting and the decision-making process in health care: Some postwar characteristics of health policy in Sweden) (Ph.D. diss., University of Uppsala, Sweden, 1989).

9. Richard B. Saltman, "Emerging Trends in the Swedish Health System," *International Journal of Health Services* 21 (1991): 625–23.

10. Lennarth Johansson and Mats Thorslund, "Care Needs and Sources of Support in a Nationwide Sample of Elderly in Sweden," *Zeitschrift für Gerontologie* 25, no. 1 (1992): 57–62.

11. Baldock and Evers, "Innovations"; Julia Twigg, "The Interweaving of Formal and Informal Care: Policy Models and Problems," in Evers and van der Zanden, *Better Care for Dependent People Living at Home,* pp. 115–32.

12. OECD, "Financing and Delivering Health Care—a Comparative Analysis of OECD Countries," in *OECD Social Policy Studies,* vol. 4 (Paris: OECD, 1987); OECD, "Health Care Systems in Transition: The Search for Efficiency," in *OECD Social Policy Studies,* vol. 7 (Paris: OECD, 1990).

13. Mats Thorslund and Marti G. Parker, "Strategies for an Ageing Population: Expanding the Priorities Discussion," *Ageing and Society* 15 (1995) (forthcoming).

14. Mats Thorslund, "Äldres Flyttningar till Service och Vård" (Admissions of elderly people to institutions and special housing), *Ädelutvärderingen* 93, no. 9 (Stockholm: National Board of Health and Welfare, 1993), pp. 7–45; Martha Szebehely, *Hemtjänst eller Anhörigvård? Förändringar under 80-talet* (Home services for elderly persons or their families? Changes during the eighties) (Stockholm: National Board of Health and Welfare, 1993); Mårten Lagergren, "De-institutionalization and Ageing: Some Results from Monitoring the Effects in an Area-Based System of Long-Term Care for Elderly People and People with Disabilities," *Health and Social Care* 2 (1994): 19–30.

15. Health Services Commission, *Prioritized List of Health Services* (Portland, Oregon: Health Services Commission, 1992).

16. NOU, *Retningslinjer for Prioritering innen Norsk Helsevesen* (Guidelines for setting priorities in Norwegian health care) (Oslo: Ministry of Social Affairs, 1987).

17. The Government Committee on Choices in Health Care, *Choices in Health Care* (Rijswijk, Netherlands: Ministry of Welfare, Health, and Cultural Affairs, 1992).

18. SOU, *Vårdens Svåra Val: Rapport från Utredningen om Prioriteringar inom Hälso- och sjukvården* (Difficult choices in health care: Report concerning setting of priorities in medical care) (Stockholm: Ministry of Social Affairs, 1993).

19. A. J. Culyer, *Health Care and Health Care Finance in Sweden: The Crisis That Never Was, the Tensions That Ever Will Be,* Occasional Paper 33 (Stockholm: SNS, November 1991).

Ruud H. J. ter Meulen

Solidarity with the Elderly and the Allocation of Resources

One of the cornerstones of European health care systems is the principle of solidarity. The care of the elderly, including health care and social care, is in many respects based on this principle: the young contribute to the costs of care for the old, who have a greater risk of disease and handicaps. But the increasing demand for care by the elderly—resulting from epidemiological changes as well as various social processes—is putting solidarity between the young and the old under strain. Particularly the medicalization of old age, which is draining away resources from long-term care, is an important threat to the preparedness of the younger generations to take care of the needs of older persons. One of the theses of this essay is that the process of medicalization should be stopped, not by an age limit (as advocated by Daniel Callahan and others) but by introducing a two-tier system based on the principle of humanitarian solidarity.

Longer Life, Worsening Health

Since the beginning of this century, the average life expectancy has risen significantly in the industrialized world. In the early 1900s, it was approximately fifty years. At this moment, the average life expectancy is seventy-six years for both the United States and for the member states of the European Community (EC). Life expectancy is higher for women than for men: seventy-three for men and seventy-nine years for women in the EC. The increase of the average life expectancy is expected to continue: in the year 2025 it will be eighty years, seventy-seven years for men and eighty-two years for women.[1]

The increase of average life expectancy, however, cannot be called a success in all respects.[2] While individuals can enjoy themselves in a longer life, they are suffering from chronic, debilitating diseases that are typical for the later stages of life. The higher one's age, the greater the risk of being handicapped by chronic diseases, for example, diseases of the sensory organs or neurological and cardiovascular diseases. In fact, the *healthy* life expectancy, that is, the period of life that is free from diseases and handicaps, has remained the same, but the *average* life expectancy has risen. Consequently, we are living in bad health for an increasing part of our lives.[3]

Noting the difference between healthy life expectancy and average life expectancy, we can understand better the increasing demand for long-term care. This is particularly true for the age-group eighty years and above, the fastest growing age-group in the industrialized world: from 16 million in the EC in 1980 to 29 million in 2010.[4] This age-group is particularly tortured physically and psychologically by dementia, depression, osteoporosis (including the breaking of hips and arms), and cerebral-vascular accidents. Moreover, the eighty-year-olds have an increasing chance for lesser but not less debilitating handicaps, such as visual and acoustic impairments, genitourinary diseases, and psychiatric disorders. They are also afflicted by loneliness, social abandonment, and poor nutrition.[5] As a result of these handicaps, the eighty-year-olds are, more than any other age-group, dependent on professional care, particularly home care, nursing home care, and hospital care. The rapid growth of this age-group will result in a sharp rise in the demand for care in the near future.

Social Processes and the Demand for Care

In light of demographic projections and epidemiological developments, how large will be the increase in the demand for care by the elderly? There is no easy answer to this question: the demand for care is determined not solely by demographic process but by other social processes as well.[6] The most important of these processes are medicalization, decreasing availability of informal care, and the values and norms attached to old age.

Medicalization can be defined as the process by which human existence is increasingly understood in terms of health and disease,[7] and it is characterized by an increasing utilization of medical services. This will very likely continue to increase in the coming decades because of the continuous growth of medical knowledge on the one hand and the increasing public awareness of the possibilities of this technology on the other hand.[8] Patients and doctors are moved by a "quest for certainty," which is very costly, as more and more diagnostics have to be performed to rule out disease or to confirm a diagnosis.

The *availability of informal care*—care given by family members or neighbors—also affects the level of demand for medical care. As a result of the ongoing individualization of society and the breakdown of traditional forms of solidarity, this kind of informal care is becoming scarcer. Children are moving away from their parents to other cities, having their own families, or getting divorced. They have a more individualistic lifestyle with norms and values that are different from those of their elder parents. Moreover, an increasing part of the population is living in arrangements other than the traditional family. The willingness to provide informal care is also lessened by a decline in the number of children and the emancipation of women. Moreover, at the same time that parents are becoming needy, their children are already at an age at which they likely will have problems with their own health. Instead of burdening children or neighbors, the elderly are more inclined to ask for professional help.

The *values and norms attached to old age* are also playing an important role in the demand for care. Though the elderly are very often willing to work longer and to make themselves useful for society, they are forced to leave the workforce at the age of sixty-five or even earlier. Because employment opportunities will not likely increase in the future (partly because of the increasing participation of women), the pensioning age will probably not be changed in the coming decades. In general, the elderly are expected to disengage from society, making room for younger generations.

It can be expected that the difference between the aspirations of the elderly, on the one hand, and the unwillingness of society to respond to these aspirations on the other, will result in lower responsibility for health and a decline in subjective health status. These processes will give rise to increasing visits to general practitioners and to an increasing utilization of other medical services.

Scarcity of Care Resources

For the Netherlands, it is expected that as a result of the demographic process only (that is, the increase of the number of aged and very aged persons, combined with their mortality rates and their objective and subjective health status), the demand for care will increase at the rate of 1 percent each year.[9] This figure can be lower or higher, depending on the degree of influence of social processes mentioned above.

Increasing medicalization and individualization and the worsening of the position of the elderly in society will result in a faster increase in the demand for care. For the Netherlands, the figure will then be more than the 1 percent, which is predicted for the demographic shift alone. If the medicalization decreases and the solidarity between the generations increases, then the demand for care will decrease and will be less than 1 percent. It is expected, however, that the former, not the latter, scenario will take place. In the Netherlands, and probably also in other Western European countries, we will have to reckon with an increase in the demand for care at a rate of probably 3 or 4 percent each year.

Opposed to this increasing demand for care is a decreasing willingness of national governments to enlarge the share of health care in the gross national product. More money for health care results in less collective spending on other social activities and services, such as education, environmental care, public housing, and road construction. Some of these services are as important for good health as health care specifically. An upward pressure from the rising costs of health care on individual incomes (by means of insurance premiums or out-of-pocket payments) is not desirable either, as it will endanger the solidarity between the higher and the lower income groups, which is one of the pillars of European health care systems.

There is another argument for limitation of resources for health care. More money will not satisfy the demand for care. Medical technology will always produce new devices for the diagnosis or cure of diseases. These devices are immediately claimed by the patients or their doctors as a right. The scarcity of health care resources is a structural problem that is tightly linked to our culture and our way of life, in which health and health care play a dominant role.[10] More money for health care will not result in less demand for care.

Limits to health care will result in scarce resources. The Dutch government, for example, has decided that the yearly increase of resources will be no more than 1 percent. This figure is just enough to account for the increasing demand by the demographic shift only.[11] But as we have seen above, the annual demand for care will probably be much higher. Consequently, there are waiting lists for many services, particularly those for the elderly. In the Netherlands there are large waiting lists for nursing homes, homes for the elderly, home care, and cataract surgery.

Solidarity with the Elderly

Care for the elderly in most European countries is based on the principle of solidarity. Solidarity means that the strong—for example, persons with high incomes or low health risks—contribute toward the costs of the care for the weak, that is, persons with lower incomes or greater risks for diseases and handicaps. The principle of solidarity assumes the conscious and voluntary choice for unity with certain people, groups, or populations.[12] This choice was once limited to members of an individual's immediate group, for instance, family, village, or social class. This "group solidarity" played an important role in the history of health care insurance. Workers, employees, or civil servants united voluntarily in sickness funds to safeguard themselves against the financial risks of disease and physical or mental handicap. Solidarity was not limited to health insurance but was a basic principle in other social-security schemes as well, such as pensioning schemes, unemployment and disability insurance, and workers' compensation.

As society changes into a loose community of individuals or small groups protected by collective arrangements of the state, group solidarity is replaced by a solidarity of interests. Out of clear self-interest, people are now sharing certain risks together with individuals belonging to other social categories. Such solidarity is not a conscious choice for unity with people in the same group but a compulsory measure enforced by the state. Nowadays solidarity means the obligation to share the financial risks of illness and handicap with other people not necessarily of one's own social group. In exchange for meeting the obligation to pay a premium, people have access to a broad package of health care services.

Solidarity of interests is based on the principle of reciprocity: people share risks that are common to each other. For uncommon risks or risks that are the result of irresponsible behavior, there is only a narrow base. In an era of limited resources, general solidarity across groups is giving way to a tendency to blame groups of persons who are limiting the access to care services by their irresponsible behavior or excessive health claims. Public attention is focused on persons who put their health at risk by unhealthy lifestyles or dangerous activities, particularly people who smoke, drink, use drugs, engage in unprotected sex, or injure themselves by playing sports. According to this view, these persons ought to be limited in their access to health care services because of their lack of responsible behavior. But the reason these groups of persons are blamed or discriminated against is often arbitrary; there are many activities that are dangerous or have health risks.[13] Blaming some groups for the scarcity of resources is a kind of scapegoating, which has often to do with prejudice and moralism.

It is not unlikely that the elderly will be victimized in the same way. Historically, attitudes toward the elderly have never been positive and will inevitably become more negative in times of scarce resources. Because of their increasing demand for care and their dependency on others, the elderly are seen as more and more of a burden for society. They occupy an increasing number of beds within the hospitals, which in some cases results in waiting lists for younger patients. Premiums for health care insurance are rising to pay the increasing costs of the care for the elderly. The scarcity of institutional care and home care is putting pressure on families and neighbors to take care of their elderly family members.

For their part, the elderly react with feelings of powerlessness and superfluity. This is particularly true in the Central European countries, where respect for the elderly is already low and will deteriorate further as they impose more burdens on society and their families. The same process is also true for Western European countries—for example, the United Kingdom, where the social status of the elderly is rapidly declining, partly because of their rising demand for care. The growing phenomenon of elderly abuse in nearly all European countries is writing on the wall.[14] Besides, the elderly have the idea that they are discriminated against, covertly or even overtly (as, for example, happens in the British National Health System). Organizations of Dutch elderly point out that the majority of waiting lists are for services that are important for the elderly, such as nursing home care, home care, cataract surgery, and hip replacements.

It would not be fair to blame the elderly for the scarcity of resources (as seems to be done in some countries). The demographic shift is only partly responsible for the growing demand for health care. Much more important is the impact of medicalization and individualization and the decrease in solidarity between the generations. The increase in the number and proportion of the elderly in the population is not the main cause of the growing demand for care; it is, rather, the way the elderly are treated by our society in general and the medical system in particular.[15] The rise in demand for care has much to do with high and exaggerated expectations of medicine's potential to enlarge the quality and quantity of our lives. The alleged impact of demography on the demand for care is thus grossly exaggerated: focusing on the demographic process looks very much like creating a myth, which hinders an insight into the real causes of the scarcity of resources. The elderly are an easy target who by their alleged excessive claim on health care are said to be limiting the access to care for other age-groups.

Medicalization of Old Age

Without blaming the victim, we must still rethink our solidarity across generations. The increasing demand for care by the elderly is putting heavy strains on the social resources for health care and on the willingness of younger generations to take care of their dependent parents. Are the elderly entitled to all of our resources for health care, or may we set some limits on what care they will receive?

This problem emerges particularly in acute-care medicine. There is a tendency to treat older and older patients with sophisticated medical technologies.[16] The number of people over eighty years or even ninety years of age who are getting open-heart surgery, organ transplantation, or renal dialysis is increasing rapidly. These medical treatments do not simply prolong organic life but are really beneficial in restoring health and quality of life. Octogenarians, for example, are benefiting very well from open-heart surgery. A leading Dutch cardiologist said recently that "age is hardly an indication against cardiac surgery for patients who are in a good condition."[17] In fact, the real "problem" is that a growing number of elderly are in very good condition and eligible for nearly all kinds of medical interventions, even in their eighties or nineties.

This medicalization of old age, which is driven by the dynamics of health care economics, will put increasing strains on intergenerational solidarity in two ways. First, it will hinder the access of younger patients to acute-care services. This is already apparent in the field of heart transplantation, where there is a structural scarcity of donor organs—that is, the scarcity is the result not of financial resources (so that it could be removed by greater efficiency or more money) but of other social or physical causes. The same problem is coming up in intensive-care units: though the elderly benefit from high-technology procedures, they need more time to recover in the intensive-care unit. The "greying" of these units will result in limited access of younger persons who are in extreme need. For instance, in December 1990 a young child died in Amsterdam because there was no room in the ICUs of the hospitals of the neighboring city of Haarlem, which were in large part occupied by elderly patients.

A second problem is that the increased use of acute-care services will drain away resources from long-term care. Consequently, there will be a growing demand for informal care by family members or neighbors. Though many of them, particularly daughters, are willing to supply this care, there are limits to their physical and emotional resources. While most adult children want to express solidarity with their own parents, they do have their own life plans and their own children to care for.

Limits on the Elderly?

One of the most hotly debated proposals in the ethics of resource allocation is the notion of setting an age limit for acute-care services. Well known (and controversial) are the ideas of Daniel Callahan, who opposes the medicalization of old age and believes that within the next twenty to thirty years, it may be necessary to set an age limit on the use of expensive, life-prolonging technology.[18] He proposes instead that the emphasis be given to providing decent economic support and long-term and home care. There should be, that is, a shift from curing to caring beyond a certain age (he suggests the late seventies or early eighties as the time to draw the line), with the goal of ensuring a good balance of resources between young and old and a limit to efforts to push back endlessly the frontiers of acute-care medicine for the old.

This proposal for the allocation of resources for the elderly has been strongly criticized as a kind of "ageist" discrimination.[19] Gerontologists and liberal ethicists particularly have argued that every age has its own aims and that nobody can determine for another whether his life is completed or his "natural life span" has been reached. There is no reason, they argue, to suppose that an old person values his life less than a younger one. When one considers only years of life instead of life only, one shows no respect for the unique value of the human person, which is the moral basis for our society.

Other authors have doubts about the financial savings of Callahan's proposal. The increase of health care expenditures that come with age is due not to life-extending treatments but largely to visits to general practitioners and hospitalization.[20] Regarding hospital care for the elderly, most admissions for the elderly are for life-enhancing care, that is, care that tries to improve those physical functions that are needed for normal daily activities.[21] At the end of life, the largest share of the costs of care is taken by the care in nursing homes, home care, and other kinds of long-term care. The costs of intensive, life-extending hospital care are much lower, compared to the costs of nursing and supporting.[22] For each person, most costs of care are incurred at the end of life, particularly in the last twelve months of life. These are, however, mainly expensive labor costs for nursing and caring, with only a small portion of costs attributed to aggressive, intensive treatment for patients who are moribund.[23]

Indeed, limiting acute, life-extending care for the elderly *at this moment* will not solve the allocation problem, as there will be no (direct) financial gain. The increasing medicalization of old age, however, will result in an increasing utilization of curative services by elderly persons in the future. It is therefore expected that limits to acute cure for the elderly will in the coming decades make more of a substantial contribution to the allocation of resources for the elderly than in the present situation. Still, it must be doubted that age limits will solve the allocation problem, now or in the near future. To be sure, there are situations on a clinical level in which treatment possibilities are limited and a choice must be made between a person who had a "fair share of life" and one who has not. In such situations it would not be unreasonable to choose for the latter. Turning such decisions into an official policy, however, might reinforce a negative view of old age and the elderly in our society. In fact, this would result in a lower responsibility by the elderly for their health and a lower subjective health status. A policy of age rationing will, then, ultimately result in more visits by the elderly to physicians, particularly general practitioners, and thus contribute to an *increase* in the demand for care.

Apart from these concerns, there are serious doubts that an age criterion will ever be accepted in modern society. Part of the process of individualization, referred to above, is the disappearance of traditional social relationships. Traditional values and structures of authority are replaced by relationships based on negotiation and equal respect. This process can be noted in the clinic (doctor-patient relationship)[24] as well as in other social areas, such as the family, the school, and the workplace. Two important features of the negotiation process are that it presupposes no fixed rules or shared notions of the good and that age and generation are losing ground as criteria for social arrangements and relationships.[25] Such an "age-irrelevant" society, as Bernice Neugarten styled it, is a perfect breeding ground for liberal ideologies that deny any special status to the elderly other than that they are equal to any other person in society.

Access to Care

When there is a scarcity of resources, the better off will have more opportunities to buy a better quality of care or to jump waiting lists for scarce medical treatments. National governments, unwilling to make difficult choices in health care, are trying to increase personal financial responsibility for health care services, for instance, by copayments, compulsory deductibles, or additional private insurance. Most of these payments are for long-term care services, none of them for acute care (with an exception, in some countries, for medical drugs). This shift from collective responsibility toward private responsibility fits very well with the retreat of the welfare state, the introduction of market forces, and a greater emphasis on freedom in the health care system. More freedom will inevitably result, however, in greater inequalities in access to care. Particularly the elderly, many with low incomes and pensions, will be affected by such policies.

The introduction of such a two-tier system in health care—that is, a system with a universally accessible basic tier financed by society and, above it, a privately financed tier—is often criticized as a danger to solidarity and equality, which are basic values for European health care systems. But provided that society is supplying an adequate package of health care services to which all persons have equal access (unhindered by copayments or other financial obstacles), persons who buy their own services exceeding this package do not offend any ethical principle in doing so.[26]

An important question is, of course, What is an adequate package of care services, particularly for the elderly? The answer to this question depends on society's values and its expectations for health care. One value, which in many countries is strongly adhered to, is "humanitarian solidarity." This kind of solidarity, which is based on the dignity of the human person, wants to protect those human persons whose existence is threatened by circumstances beyond their own control, particularly natural causes or unfair social structures.[27] Humanitarian solidarity should be the starting point for defining necessary care, as was advocated by the Committee on Choices in Health Care in the Netherlands. Care services for persons unable to care for themselves because of psychological handicaps—for example, by Alzheimer's disease, psychiatric disorders, or mental retardation—should have priority in the basic package. The remaining content (and extent) of the basic package should be given over, in rank order, to other kinds of long-term care (for example, home care), acute-care services, and less important health care services. Defined in this way, the basic package should be equally accessible to all, without financial constraints such as copayments or obligatory risks. Persons wanting acute-care services not supplied by the basic package should pay those services out of their own pocket or insure themselves privately for those services.

Primacy of Care

A two-tier system based on the principle of humanitarian solidarity puts care, and not cure, at the center of its efforts to provide an adequate level of health care. While cure has a permanent tendency to vanquish the barriers of illness and death, care has much more modest aspirations and is more self-containing.[28] Moreover, the emphasis on care can preserve the respect for the human person that might be endangered by the need to set limits and by the exclusion of acute services from the basic package, for example, by a two-tier system.[29] By securing access to long-term care services and limiting access to some acute-care services, a two-tier system based on the principle of humanitarian solidarity might limit the medicalization of old age, which is the most important threat to solidarity between the young and the old.

REFERENCES

1. N. Keyfitz and W. Flieger, *World Population Growth and Aging: Demographic Trends in the Late Twentieth Century* (Chicago: University of Chicago Press, 1990).

2. E. M. Gruenberg, "The Failures of Success," *Milbank Memorial Fund Quarterly/Health and Society* 55, no. 1 (Winter 1977): 3–24.

3. M. Haan et al., eds., "Living Longer and Doing Worse? Present and Future Trends in the Health of the Elderly," special issue, *Journal of Aging and Health* 3, no. 2 (1991): 133–308.

4. A. R. Taket, "Resource Allocation Problems and Health Services for the Elderly," *World Health Statistics Quarterly* 45 (1992): 89–94.

5. D. Hamerman and A. Fox, "Responses of the Health Professions to the Demographic Revolution: A Multidisciplinary Perspective," *Perspectives in Biology and Medicine* 35 (1992): 583–93.

6. C. F. Hollander and H. A. Becker, eds., *Growing Old in the Future: Scenarios in Health and Aging, 1984–2000* (Dordrecht: Nijhoff, 1987).

7. I. K. Zola, "Medicine as an Institution of Social Control," *Sociological Review* 20 (1972): 487–504.

8. Paul J. van der Maas, "Aging and Public Health," in *Health and Aging: Perspectives and Prospects,* ed. J. J. F. Schroots et al. (Lisse, The Netherlands: Swets and Zietlinger, 1988), pp. 95–115.

9. J. Naaborg, "Benodigde en beschikbare middelen, een groeiend probleem voor de zorgverlening" (Required and available resources, an increasing problem in the delivery of health care), in Commissie Keuzen in de Zorg, *Kiezen en delen: Rapport van de Commissie Keuzen in de Zorg* (Government committee on choices in health care, Choosing and sharing: report of the committee on choices in health care), part 2, Achtergrondstudies (Rijwijk, the Netherlands: Ministerie van WVC, 1991), chap. 4.

10. Daniel Callahan, *What Kind of Life: The Limits of Medical Progress* (New York: Simon and Schuster, 1990).

11. Government Committee on Choices in Health Care, *Choices in Health Care* (Rijswijk, Netherlands: Ministry of Welfare, Health, and Cultural Affairs, 1992).

12. Government Committee on Choices in Health Care, *Choices in Health Care,* p. 56.

13. D. Wikler, "Personal Responsibility for Illness," in *Health Care Ethics,* ed. D. Vanderveer and T. Regan (Philadelphia: Temple University Press, 1987), pp. 326–58.

14. N. Everaerts, J. Peraer, and I. Ponjaert-Kristoferson, *Zorg om zorg: Misbehandelen van ouderen* (Concern for care: Mistreatment of elderly persons) (Leuven/Apeldoorn: Garant, 1993).

15. P. G. Clark, "Canadian Health-Care Policy and the Elderly: Will Rationing Rhetoric Become Reality in an Aging Society?" *Canadian Journal of Community Mental Health* 8 (1989): 123–40.

16. Daniel Callahan, "Setting Limits: A Response," *Gerontologist* 34, no. 3 (1994): 393–98.

17. R. W. Koster, "Cardiologie bij ouderen" (Cardiology with the elderly), in *Ouder worden nu '90* (Aging now '90), ed. C. P. M. Knipscheer, J. J. M. Michels, and M. W. Ribbe (Alemere: Versluys, 1990), pp. 311–15.

18. Daniel Callahan, *Setting Limits: Medical Goals in an Aging Society* (New York: Simon and Schuster, 1987).

19. See, for example, Robert H. Binstock and Stephen G. Post, eds., *Too Old for Health Care? Controversies in Medicine, Law, Economics, and Ethics* (Baltimore: Johns Hopkins University Press, 1991). See the rebuttal by Callahan to these and other criticisms in "Setting Limits: A Response."

20. H. de Jouvenel, *Europe's Ageing Population: Trends and Challenges to 2025* (Guildford: Butterworths, 1989).

21. For example, the most often performed operations for the elderly in Dutch hospitals are cataract surgery, prostate surgery, hip replacement, and treatment for inguinal ruptures. The first life-extending treatment—coronary bypass grafting—is on line 14. On the basis of this list, the chairman of the Dutch Health Council, Mrs. Borst-Eilers, has calculated that limiting life-extending care to people over seventy-five would save only 100 to 200 million guilders, that is, equivalent to 0.5 percent of the Dutch health care budget of 40 billion guilders. See E. Borst-Eilers, "Leeftijd als criterium" (Age as criterion), in *Grenzen aan de zorg: Zorgen aan de grens,* ed. J. K. M. Gevers and H. J. Hubben (Alphen aan de Rijn: Tjeenk Willink, 1990), pp. 66–72.

22. D. Jahnigen and R. H. Binstock, "Economic and Clinical Realities: Health Care for Elderly People," in Binstock and Post, *Too Old for Health Care?* pp. 13–43.

23. A. A. Scitovsky, "The High Cost of Dying: What Do the Data Show?" *Milbank Memorial Fund Quarterly* 62, no. 4 (1984): 591–608; A. A. Scitovsky and A. M. Capron, "Medical Care at the End of Life: The Interaction of Economics and Ethics," *Annual Review of Public Health* 7 (1986): 59–78; A. A. Scitovsky, "Medical Care in the Last Twelve Months of Life: The Relation between Age, Functional Status, and Medical Expenditures," *Milbank Memorial Fund Quarterly* 66, no. 4 (1988): 640–60.

24. Harry R. Moody, "From Informed Consent to Negotiated Consent," *Gerontologist* 28, supplement (1988): 64–70.

25. Harry R. Moody, "The Meaning of Life and the Meaning of Old Age," in *What Does It Mean to Grow Old? Reflections from the Humanities,* ed. Thomas R. Cole and Sally A. Gadow (Durham: Duke University Press, 1986), pp. 9–40.

26. President's Commission for the Study of Ethical Problems in Medicine and Biomedical and Behavioral Research, *Securing Access to Health Care: A Report on the Ethical Implications of Differences in the Availability of Health Services* (Washington: U.S. Government Printing Office, 1983), p. 20.

27. Government Committee Choices in Health Care, *Choices in Health Care,* p. 57.

28. Callahan, *What Kind of Life?,* p. 145.

29. Ibid., p. 149.

BRYAN JENNETT

The Elderly and High-Technology Therapies

There are conflicting signals about the benefits and burdens of high-technology therapies for the elderly. Some are concerned that the routine application of cardiopulmonary resuscitation and intensive care for elderly patients in acute crises may serve only to prolong the dying process and deprive the patient of death with dignity. A *New England Journal of Medicine* editorial stated: "The very high suicide rate in older Americans is due partly to concern that they may be unable to stop treatment if hospitalized. Some people now fear living more than dying, because they dread becoming prisoners of technology."[1]

Others are more concerned that because of failure to recognize the benefits that treatment can bring, elderly patients may be deprived of access to therapies that could both extend and enhance their lives.[2] These advocates for the elderly emphasize that although fewer of an unselected group of elderly patients may respond well to treatment than would younger patients, many suitably selected elderly patients do well. It has been suggested that the absolute benefit to these patients is more relevant than whether such benefit is statistically less probable than for younger patients.[3] Such advocates counsel against age as a selection faction per se, pointing out that the proper influence of age is as a marker for factors that may adversely affect outcome, such as reduced physiological reserve and comorbidity. These factors, not age itself, should affect the decision whether treatment is likely to be worthwhile. Decision makers may also believe that the reduced expectation of life of older persons greatly limits the benefit that comes from rescuing the patient from a life-threatening illness. In fact the expectation of life in patients who have already survived to sixty-five years or more is considerably greater than is often realized, while the extension of life resulting from active therapeutic intervention can make this well worthwhile.[4] In spite of these concerns that the elderly may sometimes be unfairly deprived of access to various types of high technology, the evidence is that in both the United States and the United Kingdom, the elderly form a considerable proportion of those receiving various high technologies (table 1); moreover this proportion is tending to increase year by year.

TABLE 1

Percentage of Elderly (over Sixty-Five) in the United States

Of the total population (1980)	11%
On dialysis	31%
Receiving resuscitation	55%
Receiving ventilation	34%
Receiving artificial nutrition	48%
Of those on nasogastric tube	53%
Of those on intravenous tube	40%
Intensive-care-unit admissions	44%

Percentage of Elderly (over Sixty-Five) in the United Kingdom

Of the total population	14%
Receiving surgical operations	22%
Surgical admissions	25%
Urology/Ophthalmology admissions	50%
In general intensive-care unit	31% (24%–46%)
Receiving coronary care	52%

In analyzing the dilemma of which technologies are appropriate for which elderly patients, it is helpful to identify different types of technology and the kinds of patients who might benefit from them. Therapeutic technologies fall into three categories. First are those that are lifesaving, such as cardiopulmonary resuscitation, emergency surgery, intensive care, and dialysis. Some of these also feature in the second category, those that are life-sustaining—for example, dialysis, mechanical ventilation, and tube feeding. The third category of technologies are those that are life-enhancing; most are elective surgical interventions that improve quality of life. These include operations for coronary-artery disease, cataract, or prostate enlargement, as well as joint replacements and renal transplants.

Patients who may be considered for interventions that aim to save or sustain life can be categorized in different ways, which affect how decisions whether to intervene or not are made. Some patients, previously well, have had a sudden unexpected crisis—a heart attack, stroke, or head injury. In such instances an initial trial of treatment will almost always be justified to observe the response of the patient before considering whether to continue treatment. Quite different are patients with progressive disorders in whom a predictable crisis or relapse occurs and about whom some prior decision about future treatment may have been made following discussion with the patient and family. Such are patients with progressive organ failure—of heart, lungs, brain, kidneys, or liver—and those with advanced cancer or dementia. A third category comprises those, already disabled by progressive disease, who fall victim to an unpredictable accident or acute illness unrelated to their existing disease; the most common of these are severely demented patients. In each of these categories, some patients are competent and can participate in decisions about their treatment, while others cannot. The latter includes those with acute brain failure due to intracranial trauma, hemorrhage, or infection or to systemic disease affecting cerebral function, as well as those with chronic dementia.

Decisions to initiate or continue with technologies that save or sustain life in patients of any age should depend on balancing the expected benefits and possible burdens of intervention, and on the patient's preference. This preference can be properly exercised only if the patient is fully informed about the implications of various treatment options. Intervention may be deemed inappropriate if it is unwanted by the patient or his surrogates, after explanation about its likely effect. It may, however, be unfair even to offer such treatment as an option if it is considered that no benefit is likely to be derived from treatment—either because the severity of illness is such that there is unlikely to be a favorable response to treatment or that at best it will only briefly postpone a fatal outcome. Doctors, however, need to guard against withholding treatment on too ready an assumption that patients would not consider some limited relief of symptoms and extension of life worthwhile, because the perceptions and aspirations of the elderly themselves may differ from those of younger people, including their doctors and families. Doctors need also to guard against deciding to withhold treatment on grounds of limited resources while implying that the decision is based on a belief that treatment is not clinically indicated.[5]

Nonetheless there is good evidence that patients of all ages are frequently overtreated, particularly those who present with critical illness requiring emergency surgery, resuscitation, or intensive care. The most common reason doctors do this is ignorance about the probability of benefit for a patient of a particular age and severity of illness. There may be a lack of available data, which is particularly true for the elderly because, even for conditions for which good trial data have been produced, entry to such trials has often excluded the elderly. There may be published data that are unknown to the decision maker, but more often he or she chooses to ignore known data. This may be because of pressures from other doctors, nurses, and relatives who seem to expect intervention rather than watchful waiting. It may be that the doctor is unwilling to face the hopelessness of the situation and the futility of intervention. Sometimes a decision to embark on a trial of treatment is well justified, but it may not be explicitly defined as such to the therapeutic team and to the family. If this has been explained at the outset, it is likely to be easier to withdraw treatment once it is evident that no useful response has been observed. Unless there is a willingness to withdraw treatment that is proving of no benefit, some doctors may be reluctant to initiate potentially beneficial treatment for fear of being left committed to a period of futile support if the patient does not respond well. This applies particularly to elderly patients who may reasonably be given the opportunity to benefit from surgery or intensive care, but only with a prior agreement that if complications develop or there is not an immediate good response, further treatment will be abandoned. This issue for the elderly has been explored with reference to prolonged ventilation in particular,[6] and to catastrophic situations in general.[7]

Given these generalizations about the factors that influence decisions regarding use of therapeutic technologies for the elderly, a number of specific technologies that provoke controversy are now described to illustrate the dilemmas of decision making more clearly.

Intensive Care

Patients over sixty-five years of age account for between a quarter and a half of most ICU admissions, and there is considerable variation in the reported influence of age on outcome.[8] In a review of six units in the United Kingdom, three showed no difference in mortality between the patients over and under age sixty-five; in the other three the elderly did much worse (table 2).[9] It is likely that admission policies may have excluded those with obviously poor prognosis from the first three units. Other reports, correcting for severity of illness by the APACHE II formula, found that patients over seventy-five had no worse ICU mortality than fifty-five- to sixty-five-year-olds but did have a higher hospital mortality.[10] When later mortality (up to two years) is considered, age has a marked effect,[11] although others have reported that the mortality rate at six months is similar to that of a healthy age-matched population.[12] No difference was found in the one-year mortality or in quality of life measures at one, six, and twelve months after discharge between patients over seventy-five and those in the next lower decade in another report.[13]

These somewhat conflicting results are probably explained by variations in case mix, with some series having diagnostic restrictions, such as exclusion of cases of malignancy. It seems apparent, however, that chronic illness before the acute crisis is an important predictor of later mortality in those who survive critical care, while precrisis quality of life is a good predictor of restoration to a good quality of life.[14] All seem agreed that what matters is not chronological age but biological age; there are, however, no good markers for the latter other

TABLE 2 Elderly in United Kingdom Intensive-Care Units

United Kingdom Hospitals	Number of Patients	Proportion of Admissions over Sixty-Five	Mortality Rates for under Sixty-Five	Mortality Rates for over Sixty-Five
A	432	24%	27%	23%
B	693	25%	22%	24%
C	606	38%	14%	17%
D	215	29%	20%	39%
E	401	46%	10%	26%
F	693	26%	5%	28%

Source: B. Jennett, "The Elderly and High Technology Therapies," in *Health Problems of an Ageing Population,* ed. N. Wells and C. Freer (London: Macmillan, 1988).

than the presence or absence of established progressive disease. A limitation of many of these studies is that they compare outcome in patients over sixty-five or over seventy-five with patients in the next younger decade. But many studies have shown that the relationship between mortality and increasing age is continuous over many years, without any watershed at any particular age. It is therefore not surprising that differences between one decade and the next are not very great. It would seem, however, that age has a limited influence on early mortality in patients needing intensive care and that a trial of treatment is well justified in patients who have APACHE scores indicating a reasonable expectation of survival and who, before becoming critically ill, were enjoying good health and quality of life. A study of patients and their relatives after intensive care (most of them over sixty-five years of age) revealed that 70 percent would be willing to undergo intensive care again, even to achieve one month's survival.[15] It may therefore be that doctors overestimate the burdens of intensive care and underestimate how much patients value even limited benefits.

Surgery

Elderly patients make up a large proportion of surgical patients, particularly in some specialties such as orthopedics, urology, and ophthalmology. The benefits of joint replacement, prostate resection, and cataract removal in enhancing quality of life are beyond dispute. In the United Kingdom surgeons admit to hospital each year more patients over seventy-five years of age than do geriatricians and internists combined. A Finnish study of 17,000 general surgical operations found that although only 20 percent were over seventy years of

TABLE 3   All Open-Heart Surgery

	1990		1991		1992	
	Of 650	*Mortality Percentage*	*Of* 690	*Mortality Percentage*	*Of* 760	*Mortality Percentage*
<69 yrs.	49%	3.1	52%	2.7	49%	3.5
60–70 yrs.	43%	5.8	39%	5.9	39%	5.9
>70 yrs.	8%	7.0	9%	6.8	49%	5.7

Coronary-Artery Bypass Graft 1992

	Of 694	*Mortality Percentage*
<60 yrs.	52%	0.8%
>60 yrs.	48%	1.8%

Source: A Glasgow unit, personal communication.

age, these older patients accounted for 91 percent of deaths.[16] A confidential enquiry showed that 79 percent of perioperative deaths in Britain were over the age of sixty-five, although only 22 percent of operations performed were in this age-group. No one can deny that operative mortality increases with age, but that is no excuse for not considering each patient individually to assess the risk factors. Very often it is associated disease in another system that makes for high risk. In the Finnish study pulmonary embolism and cardiac complications were the most common cause of death in older patients. Emergency operations always carry a higher mortality, 37 percent compared with 8 percent for elective surgery in the Finnish study; moreover, older patients more often present as emergencies. Studies of perioperative deaths in the United Kingdom have consistently shown that some 10 percent of operations are judged to have been unjustified, most of them emergency procedures in elderly patients who were moribund before operation.

Elective cardiac surgery is of particular benefit to elderly patients, who do well both after bypass grafting and valve replacement. Patients over sixty years of age now make up half of all cases of open-heart surgery in the United Kingdom, and although mortality is almost double that in the younger patients, it is still acceptably low (table 3). In deciding about cardiac (and other) surgery in the elderly, it is important to assess carefully the balance of benefits likely to come from surgery, even when age is advanced and risk seems high. A recent detailed discussion of this point used the example of an eighty-seven-year-old woman with severe aortic stenosis, three-vessel coronary-artery disease, and moderate heart failure. Her excess mortality was estimated to be 50 percent per year without surgery and 2 percent per year after successful surgery; the risks of aortic-valve replacement and coronary-bypass grafting were estimated as 11 percent mortality and 7 percent morbidity. The conclusion was that life expectancy was 5.1 years with surgery and 1.6 years without, a gain of four quality-adjusted life years (QALYs). This critique recommended the use of decision analysis and life expectancy tables[17] to avoid underestimating the probable benefit of operating on elderly patients. A report from the Royal College of Physicians of London[18] suggests that elderly patients should have better access to coronary angioplasty and cardiac surgery.

Renal Dialysis

Renal dialysis, both a lifesaving and a life-sustaining technology, has been rationed by age to a greater or lesser extent in most countries.[19] When the program began in Seattle in 1961, the upper age limit was forty-five years, but by 1985 a third of cases nationally in the United States were over sixty-five years of age. Yet even with the nationally financed program in that country, by 1987 a patient over sixty-five was only half as likely to get dialysis as a younger patient, and for those over seventy-five the chances dropped to a third. These practices reflect the observation that older patients do less well, particularly in survival data. Thus West Germany reported a five-year survival of 45 percent for sixty- to seventy-year-olds but only 25 percent for those over seventy. The latter figure was confirmed in a U.S. study and could be regarded as quite a reasonable outcome, while another study of patients over sixty-five years of age reported higher well-being indices and more positive benefits from dialysis than in younger patients. In spite of this, another U.S. study discovered that whereas only 10 percent of fifty-five- to sixty-five-year-olds considered requesting that treatment be discontinued, this figure was 20 percent for those over sixty-five. It seems therefore that although some elderly patients recognize substantial benefits from dialysis, others consider that it is not worthwhile. Indeed, stopping dialysis accounts for about one-third of deaths in elderly patients on dialysis. Discussing withdrawal of dialysis, half of 111 U.S. nephrologists indicated that they more often withheld treatment than withdrew it, while 17 percent more often withdrew it, with the remaining physicians using equally the two approaches to limiting treatment. Most often the reason for stopping dialysis was a new disease, often a stroke, but sometimes it was because of accompanying diabetes and advanced age. Most had been on dialysis for some three years when it was stopped on request. Dialysis was most often withheld initially because of existing poor quality of life from associated conditions such as dementia or a vegetative state.

Cardiopulmonary Resuscitation (CPR)

There is considerable dispute about the appropriateness of cardiopulmonary resuscitation for elderly patients. Gillon points out that it is a violent, damaging, painful, alarming, and undignified procedure that may do no more than delay a timely death.[20] A Royal College of Physicians report claims that almost half of those recently resuscitated would not want to have it done again and that prospectively only 7 percent of elderly patients would opt for it.[21] This conflicts with a questionnaire to outpatients in Aberdeen by Robertson, 97 percent of whom said they would want CPR in their present state of health, but only 10 percent if they were senile and no longer recognized people.[22] There was no difference between the responses of patients above and below the age of sixty. A crucial question, however, is whether CPR is likely to be successful. One American report claimed that no patient over seventy survived to discharge from hospital, and that few ever became oriented.[23] It reported that one-third of hospital deaths had CPR, of which a half were over sixty-five, and that of those having CPR one-third survived the episode, but only one-third of these ever left hospital, and half of them would refuse it in the future. In another American report of 503 patients over sixty-nine years of age, only 8 percent survived to discharge, and half of these went to chronic care with added disability; less than 2 percent went home.[24] The conclusion was that for most elderly patients, resuscitation was a curse rather than a blessing and was also a misuse of resources. Guidelines were recommended to help make appropriate decisions. It seems that although do-not-resuscitate orders have been available in the United States since 1976, resuscitation is still too often resorted to routinely, although protocols for withholding treatment have been mandatory in hospitals and nursing homes since 1988. Moreover, the Patient Self-Determination Act of 1990 now requires that all patients be advised on admission to hospital or nursing home of their right to refuse treatment, to write a living will, and to appoint a proxy decision maker. It seems that in the United Kingdom the urge to resuscitate is more often resisted, especially in geriatric units, although a recent case reached the Ombudsman because the relatives had not been fully informed and consulted about this decision.[25] It seems clear that a decision not to resuscitate should be based not on age alone but on the likelihood of success and of benefit to the patient if survival is secured.

Tube Feeding

Tube feeding is another technology used on different scales in the United States and United Kingdom. Most British geriatricians consider that it should be initiated only for an elderly patient who has a reasonable quality of life and has sustained an illness that is expected to be recoverable. It would not normally be instituted when a chronically demented patient began to refuse normal feeding. In the United States, however, there are reports of demented patients surviving for several years after tube feeding has been initiated. The motives for such treatment are sometimes questioned, whether it is not more for the carers than for the patient.[26] It is interesting that when the *Cruzan* case went to the United States Supreme Court for a decision about discontinuing tube feeding, the American Geriatric Society submitted an amicus curiae brief in favor of allowing the tube feeding to be stopped. Their concern was that if the Court decided not to allow tube feeding to be stopped in this young vegetative patient, there could be serious implications for the compassionate care of the elderly. Such a judgment might be read as requiring geriatricians to prolong life by tube feeding regardless of the quality of life or the hazards and discomfort of such feeding, which can be considerable in the elderly.[27]

Making Decisions about Technology for the Elderly

What factors should be considered when deciding whether to initiate or continue technologies that save or sustain life? For the most part the factors to consider are the same at all ages. Most important is the balance between the benefits and burdens of alternative management options. The doctor's role is to determine the prognosis and set out the therapeutic options, to discover the views of patient, family, and other caregivers, and then to make a decision in the light of these discussions. He or she should consider primarily the interests of the patient, but with a mind also to those of the family, caregivers, and competing patients.

In determining prognosis, there is no denying that age does influence the expected outcome of critical illness, for several reasons. One is the limited physiological reserve in various organs, another the increased likelihood of multiple pathology in older patients. A major factor influencing the outcome of surgery in the elderly is the extent and severity of disease in systems other than the one requiring treatment by surgery. Functional reserve in organ systems deteriorates from the midthirties onward, to some extent, in all people, but a feature of older patients is a greater variation between individuals in this regard. Thus it is important not to be overinfluenced by chronological age but to try to make an individualized assessment both of physiological status and of associated disease. With appropriate selection using these parameters, good results are often reported after major interventions in the elderly.

Another factor is the way in which the elderly may differ in their preferences for major technological interventions. Some elderly patients face the possibility of death with equanimity and may say that they have had enough good innings and don't wish for aggressive treatment. On the other hand, some are willing to accept higher risks of mortality from intervention than might younger patients. Yet others, confronted with the possibility of survival after treatment with a considerably reduced quality of life, are pleased to extend their lives on terms that might be unacceptable to a younger patient. It is therefore unwise to predict which way individual patients will react to the risks and benefits associated with interventions. They can make informed choices only if adequately informed by their doctors about the probabilities associated with various treatment options. Many elderly patients, however, are not competent to make their preferences known. Only occasionally is there likely to be an advance directive in the form either of a living will or of an appointed proxy decision maker, although it is hoped that these will become more common in the future. Without such a directive the doctor is left to consult with family members before deciding whether or not to treat. From their previous knowledge of the patient, the family may feel able to say how they believe this patient would wish to be treated (substituted judgment). Alternatively, the doctor and the family are left to judge on objective terms what would appear to be in this patient's best interests.

Some guidance on how people feel about such decisions comes from asking them about what they would want in a number of imagined future scenarios, as was done for five hundred outpatients and members of the public in the United States.[28] As expected, most patients elected to forgo lifesaving and life-sustaining treatment if they were vegetative or affected by advanced dementia. What was more surprising was that more than half would forgo such treatment if in a coma with a small chance of good recovery. That was also an opinion given by a number of neurosurgeons when asked about treatment after a severe head injury: they wanted treatment withdrawal at a much lower probability of poor outcome if they themselves were the patient than they would apply to their patients.[29] These studies show not only the fear of a poor-quality survival but a realization that decisions depend on probabilities, not certainties.

Decisions to limit treatment are now commonplace. A report from intensive-care units in San Francisco recently indicated that about half the deaths followed such decisions,[30] and a similar proportion was discovered in a study of surgical deaths in Scotland and in a study of deaths in Holland.[31] Many situations are relatively stereotyped, and reaching these decisions can be facilitated by having a set of guidelines that have been agreed upon by doctors and nurses in a hospital or in a clinical unit, with or without advice from an ethics committee. Most such decisions should be reached together by the doctor, the patient, and the family. When, however, there is disagreement either among the professionals or family members, it may be helpful to enlist the help of an ethics committee about an individual case. Only in the exceptional circumstance of an unresolved dispute should it be necessary to seek a judicial review, with the delay and publicity that a court hearing inevitably involves.

Decisions to use expensive and potentially hazardous technology should be made on the best information available about expected benefits and burdens and about the patient's preferences, expressed now or previously or on his or her behalf. Advanced age is a legitimate criterion to consider when making such a judgment, but doctors should ensure that they do not deny useful treatment because of arbitrary age criteria. But neither should they routinely recommend treatment for elderly patients to avoid the trouble of defending a compassionate and sensible decision to withhold or withdraw treatment.

REFERENCES

1. M. Angell, "Prisoners of Technology: The Case of Nancy Cruzan," *New England Journal of Medicine* 322 (1990): 1226–28.

2. "Do Doctors Short-change Old People?" editorial, *Lancet* 342 (1993): 1–2.

3. John F. Kilner, "Age Criteria in Medicine," *Archives of Internal Medicine* 149 (1989): 2343–46.

4. J. V. Wong, D. M. Salem, and S. G. Pauker, "You Are Never Too Old," *New England Journal of Medicine* 328 (1993): 971–75.

5. T. Hope, D. Springings, and R. Crisp. " 'Not Clinically Indicated': Patients' Interests or Resources Allocation?" *British Medical Journal* 306 (1993): 379–81.

6. A. I. Goldberg, "Life Sustaining Technology and the Elderly, *Chest* (1988): 1277–82.

7. J. A. Barondess et al., "Clinical Decision-Making in Catastrophic Situations: The Relevance of Age," *Journal of the American Geriatric Society* 36 (1988): 919–37.

8. "Intensive Care for the Elderly," editorial, *Lancet* 337 (1991): 209–10.

9. Bryan Jennett, "The Elderly and High Technology Therapies," in *Health Problems of an Ageing Population*, ed. N. Wells and C. Freer (London: Macmillan, 1988), pp. 177–90.

10. A. W. Wu, M. R. Rubin, and M. J. Rosen, "Are Elderly People Less Responsive to Intensive Care?" *Journal of the American Geriatric Society* 38 (1990): 621–27.

11. S. Ridley et al., "Long-Term Survival after Intensive Care?" *British Medical Journal* 301 (1990): 1127–30.

12. B. Zaren and R. Bergstrom, "Survival Compared to the General Population and Changes in Health Status among Intensive Care Patients," *Acta Anesthesiologica Scandinavia* 33 (1989): 6–12.

13. L. Chelluri et al., "Long-Term Outcome of Critically Ill Elderly Patients Requiring Intensive Care," *JAMA* 269 (1993): 3119–23.

14. A. Yimmon, A. Zimran, and C. Hershko, "Quality of Life and Survival Following Intensive Medical Care," *Quarterly Journal of Medicine* 71 (1989): 347–57.

15. M. Danis et al., "Patients' and Families' Preferences for Medical Intensive Care," *JAMA* 260 (1988): 797–802.

16. S. Palmberg and E. Hirsjarvi, "Mortality in Geriatric Surgery," *Gerontology* 25 (1979): 103.

17. S. Katz et al., "Active Life Expectancy," *New England Journal of Medicine* 309 (1983): 218–24.

18. Royal College of Physicians Working Group, "Cardiological Interventions in Elderly Patients," *Journal of Royal College of Physicians (London)* 25 (1991): 197–205.

19. L. S. Rothenberg, "Withholding and Withdrawing Dialysis from Elderly ESRD Patients," part 1, "A Historical View of the Clinical Experience," and part 2, "Ethical and Policy Issues," *Geriatric Nephrology and Urology* 2 (1992): 109–17; 3 (1993): 23–41.

20. R. Gillon, "Resuscitation Policies," *Journal of Medical Ethics* 18 (1992): 115–16.

21. J. Saunders, "Who's for CPR?" *Journal of Royal College of Physicians (London)* 26 (1992): 254–55.

22. G. S. Robertson, "Resuscitation and Senility: A Study of Patients' Opinions," *Journal of Medical Ethics* 19 (1993): 104–17.

23. D. L. Schiedermayer, "The Decision to Forego CPR in the Elderly Patient," *JAMA* 260 (1988): 1096–97.

24. P. J. Podrid, "Resuscitation in the Elderly: A Blessing or a Curse?" *Annals of Internal Medicine* 111 (1989): 193–95.

25. Gillon, "Resuscitation Policies."

26. A. Norberg et al., "Ethical Conflicts in Long-Term Care of the Aged: Nutritional Problems and the Patient–Care Worker Relationship," *British Medical Journal* (1980): 377–78.

27. I. Campbell-Taylor and R. H. Fisher, "The Clinical Case against Tube Feeding in Palliative Care of the Elderly," *Journal of the American Geriatric Society* 35 (1987): 1100–14.

28. L. L. Emanuel et al., "Advance Directives for Medical Care: A Case for Greater Use," *New England Journal of Medicine* 324 (1991): 889–95.

29. P. Barlow and G. Teasdale, "Prediction of Outcome and Management of Severe Head Injury: Attitudes of Neurosurgeons," *Neurosurgery* 19 (1986): 989–91.

30. N. G. Smedira et al., "Withholding and Withdrawal of Life Support from the Critically Ill," *New England Journal of Medicine* 3 (1990): 309–14.

31. P. J. Van der Mass et al., "Euthanasia and Other Medical Decisions Concerning the End of Life," *Lancet* 338 (1991): 669–74.

GEBHARD ALLERT, GERLINDE SPONHOLZ, HELMUT BAITSCH,
AND FRIEDER KELLER

The Meaning of Old Age
Impeded by Chronic Disease

Increasing life expectancy and decreasing birthrates are responsible for a significant demographic change in the industrial nations. In Germany, the proportion
of people who are sixty years and older is about 20 percent of the total
population; this is similar to other Western nations. Demographic projections
show that by the year 2025 about one-third of our population will be over
sixty. Already by the year 2000, Germany will have the highest rate of people
over sixty compared with the other European countries, the United States,
Canada, and Japan.[1]

This tremendous increase in the number of elderly people in the coming
decades will be accompanied by an even more dramatic increase in the number
of old people disabled by chronic diseases and disorders. Aside from infirmity
resulting from chronic diseases such as diabetes, heart disease, and so on, the
number of people with depression and dementia will highly increase. This is
especially the case for primary degenerative dementia, such as Alzheimer's
disease, but also vascular dementia, resulting from multiple cardiac infarctions
and such.[2] Insofar as chronic diseases such as heart diseases and diabetes are
often treated by expensive, high-tech medical procedures like bypass operations
and pump system implantations, they entail high follow-up costs as well.

Today, because of medical progress, people with chronic diseases, multi-
morbidity conditions, genetic disorders, or other primary handicaps generally
have an increased life expectancy. Since progress in medicine improves the
survival time of a growing number of chronically ill people, we are confronted
with a cost spiral of progress. This is especially true if patients have additional
age-related disabilities and health restrictions. In the ongoing passionate debate
about allocation of limited resources, the issue of health care costs for the
elderly and chronically ill becomes an increasingly virulent topic.

While the number of elderly and those in need of long-term care will
increase in the coming decades, the number of younger people responsible for
the practical care services and the financing of the needed health care will

clearly decrease. In addition, shifts in the family structure—such as the change from a three- to a two-generation family, an increase of single heads of households, and an ongoing demand for working mobility—will certainly reduce the willingness and opportunities to provide home care in the future.

To this point, the churches and social-welfare organizations in Germany have played an especially strong role in the care of the elderly and the handicapped. Because of important financial restrictions, however, their activities will be reduced, but without adequate offset by the public sector. So the question of financing the rapidly increasing costs for chronic care and the necessity of introducing a new general long-term-care insurance system have become one of the most heatedly argued topics in Germany today.[3] This public debate shows quite clearly that even now those elderly hindered by chronic disease do not have a strong lobby. Given that their number will increase dramatically, it may be feared that the level of public respect for the elderly will become even more problematic. This concern is all the more disturbing when set against the background of a general shift in values in Germany as well as in other Western societies—from solicitude and beneficence to autonomy and self-realization. This fundamental shift not only influences public opinion by eroding social appreciation of long-term care; it also affects the self-esteem of the afflicted persons.

From this discussion it becomes obvious that the question of the meaning of old age impeded by chronic diseases has many dimensions and can be approached from different standpoints. Discourse about "meaning" has to deal with its constructions on different levels, depending on underlying frames of reference and value systems. In this chapter we will focus on the following three basic levels: (1) the meaning of old age in the context of the individual life story; this is closely related to (2) the meaning of disability within interpersonal relationships (families, caregivers, self-help groups) and to (3) the social significance and public estimation of old age and disability.

So the question of meaning will not be discussed by reflecting primarily on philosophical concepts of meaning but, rather, by focusing on the model of the individual life story.

"Meaning" of Old Age and the Individual Life Story

The social understanding of old age has a long history that comprises various models of meaning. In Western societies, the development of modern medicine in the late nineteenth century established on a broad scale a model that had already become known as the "deficiency model." In this model the aging person is regarded primarily from the perspective of an ongoing deterioration of his or her mental and physical abilities. Aging is seen as a continual diminishing of personal resources and activities. Compared to the adult person, small children and old people, who are "not yet" or "no longer" in full possession of their strength, are regarded as imperfect. In contrast to these deficiency models, which are based on a reductionist biological understanding of the person, other theories, especially widespread in Eastern cultures, emphasize the growth of wisdom and life experiences of the elderly.[4]

Other models, for example, the psychodynamic model of Erik H. Erikson, focus on inner conflicts and crises related to psychodynamic development and personal growth in successive life periods. Erikson distinguishes eight consecutive life periods, the last of which—mature adult age—is characterized by the conflict between integrity, on the one hand, and loathing of life and self-contempt, on the other. Integrity means the acceptance and positive evaluation of the personal life cycle, as it stands in community spirit with other peoples and cultures.[5]

Other psychoanalytically oriented authors, such as Anneliese Heigl-Evers and Franz Heigl, emphasize the problem of accepting personal limits and failure. In the last period of life, people have to cope with failed hopes, personal guilt, and loneliness. But the elderly have special resources, such as calmness, serenity, and sense of humor, as well.[6]

In assessing the variety of understandings of old age, it is obvious that the deficiency theories in particular do not take into account the great span of individual differences among the elderly. As more and more people come to pass ninety years of age, a generation gap has developed within the cohort of the elderly. In addition, there are fundamental differences in the possibilities and interests of people who belong to the same age-group. The elderly are clearly a heterogeneous group, characterized by a great variety of abilities and a plurality of personal orientations and understandings. This variety seems even more pronounced among the elderly who suffer from chronic diseases and disorders. Their life expectations and possibilities of self-fulfillment vary widely according to age and mental or physical debility, which often changes over time. Thus any exploration of the meaning of old age accompanied by chronic disease and disability must take into account the great variety of individual circumstances, perspectives, and constructions of meaning.

Our experiences in psychotherapy, psychosomatic, and medical counseling have convinced us that the meaning of certain conflicts or handicaps as well as of personal abilities and powers can be evaluated only against profound background knowledge of the individual's biography. This has its analogue in medicine, where taking a thorough case history is crucial for giving clinicians an impression of the condition, meaning, and importance of a certain symptom.

By using the concept of the "story," which has been elaborated in the domain of medical ethics by the theologian Dietrich Ritschl, the meaning of old age and chronic illness can be discussed in a very personal and concrete way.[7] Personal identity as well as subjective self and object images, which are the main sources for individual constructions of meaning, are closely related to biographical experiences. So the question of meaning is directly related to the individual life story, which is composed of a multitude of personal experiences, episodic stories, and interpersonal relationships. The personal story correlates with different metastories—that is, with narratives of the person's family, nation, religious group, and so on. These metastories mark the underlying frames of reference, which profoundly influence the personal perception and attribution of meaning. Just as the question, Who are you? can better be answered by telling stories of significant personal experiences than by giving abstract definitions, so the question of meaning asks for such a narrative answer. In this sense we can say that to ask for meaning is to ask for stories.

In self-realization and the forming of identity, the concept of the story highlights the dimension of time. Insofar as the narratives of one's past are the most valid predictors of future personal developments, the concept of the story not only is very helpful for the actual understanding of a person but also provides a framework for future scenarios of self-realization. Especially in situations of individual crisis, which require a new orientation, this concept can support the necessary decision-making process. Furthermore, within the framework of narrative, the question of meaning is not primarily based on individual skills and intellectual abilities but focuses on personal experiences in a network of relationships. The story of a person with a handicap is closely connected with those of other people—for example, the family or the caregivers—and participates in different metastories—for example, the narrative of handicapped people in our society. Because life stories are connected in different ways at different levels, the question of the meaning of old age when accompanied by chronic illness and disorder cannot be answered from a personal standpoint alone but must also reflect the meaning of chronic illness in the network of interpersonal relationships.

"Meaning" of Disability within the Net of Personal Relationships

Families

Until today, the largest proportion by far of the labor of care was performed by families—especially women in families. This is the case even when the frail elderly person receives supplemental professional care or lives in a nursing home. The impact of increased longevity on families is that the responsibility for a handicapped family member often continues over a much longer period of time. The much-deplored disintegration of family structures is thus accompanied and relativized by a chronological prolonging of more distant but nevertheless important relationships. This phenomenon must be taken into account in any discussion of intergenerational solidarity and reciprocity. The real burden of long-term care of elderly relatives who are also mentally or physically impaired cannot clearly be anticipated by the caring family members. Especially in cases of long-lasting care and a successive deterioration of the disease, there are often profound changes in the relationships and in the acceptance of the roles as caregivers. In such cases, the caregivers do not only have increasing problems integrating their professional duties with the necessary concrete care service; they are also confronted with conflicts resulting from an inner tension between feelings of responsibility and their own wishes and conceptions of self-realization. This seems to be especially true for the generation of daughters who are the main care providers in our country. The continuous full-time, long-term care of elderly relatives often overburdens the family members physically and mentally. Therefore, on-site services and new models of care and housing for the elderly must be developed. They should relieve not only the relatives but also the neighbors and professional caregivers so that they are able to develop their own interests and live their own life stories, which are closely related to, but surely not identical with, the life story of the handicapped family member.[8]

Professional Caregivers

In contrast to the family, where a kind of common narrative always exists and where the family caregivers often have an intimate knowledge of the elderly patient, the interaction between professional caregiver and patient often begins late in the life narrative. Nevertheless, the intensive care of a person requires a wide knowledge of the patient's personal restrictions and resources as well as of his or her personal preferences and norms. Again, a thorough knowledge of the elderly person's biography seems to be extremely important. This is so not only for purposes of providing sensible and supportive care to the handicapped person but also for maintaining the personal motivation and self-esteem of the caregiver. Aside from the concrete practice of care, the practice of trading life stories helps to establish a personal relationship and creates a new story between the person in need of care and the caregiver.[9]

As with the family members, only the models that also take into account the needs and problems of those who do the work will remain useful. Those who provide this care require not only greater financial incentives but also a social upgrading of their job. These requirements are closely connected with the question of a professional educational system for providers of care to the elderly and chronically ill. Compared with the professional training of nurses in acute-care medicine, the education of long-term care providers has long been neglected, and many people working in this field today still have only a very brief training. Their curriculum must include the necessary gerontological knowledge, but in addition it seems important that it focus on communication skills and personal attitudes. Understanding and reflecting on one's personal fears and emotions when confronted with aging and dying would appear to be an integral part of any humane and responsible approach to long-term care.

This is also very important for physicians working with the chronically ill, handicapped, and the elderly. They have to accept that these patients often cannot be cured, either from their chronic diseases or from their handicaps or age-related disabilities. For these persons the physician has to be a partner helping to alleviate suffering, treating mainly symptoms rather than causes of their diseases, and being present with patients and their families. For medical decision making it is often important for the physician to know the patient's individual narrative, including personal orientations, fears, hopes, and social background. This is especially true in cases that carry substantial consequences for priority setting, for example, in deciding to treat an elderly person with a severe life-threatening lung infection at home rather than in a hospital. In situations that require informed consent, it is important not only for the physician to know the patient's decision and its narrative context; the patient should also be informed about the motives and underlying frameworks of the physician's position. In this respect, confidence, appreciation, and knowledge of the patient's narrative and a certain continuity in the care relation are basic requirements for a good care relationship between patient and caregiver.

Finally, supervision facilities for the professional caregivers and special support groups for the caregiving family members could help the care providers not only to deal better with concrete medical and practical care-related situations but also to cope better with interpersonal problems and inner conflicts. Unfortunately, such facilities are rare in Germany.

Self-Help Groups

A forum for conversing with other elderly and impaired people that permits the elderly person to share not only problems related to chronic illness but also her or his individual coping strategies and resources often seems to be extremely helpful. Such a forum permits afflicted persons to develop new contacts and relationships beyond their own families. The personal engagement in a self-help group offers a sense of solidarity with others who also experience the double burden of being old and ill. The experience of sharing one's very personal narrative of illness and fragility with others who have similar narratives to tell has a positive influence on one's self-esteem and evaluation of one's own situation.

"Meaning" of Old Age and Disability in the Macroperspective of Society

Up to now, the growing number of elderly people impeded by chronic diseases and disorders has not been a main target group of political and societal appreciation and interest in Germany. The chronically ill do not typically belong to the group of active elderly people who, on retiring from their jobs, are engaged in science, travel, culture, and politics. For this reason, the significance to society of the frail elderly cannot adequately be estimated by focusing primarily on high performance and public activity.

The concept of story, however, is useful in this context. It allows for the great variety of meanings among people afflicted with chronic disease by focusing especially on the network of relationships among the persons involved and on the correlations of individual narratives with various metanarratives. In contrast to biological-deficiency models, the story concept acknowledges that the individual's personal narrative is a source of integrity and identity, the objects of personal respect and dignity.

When we recall Germany's dreadful history of euthanasia in the Nazi era, we are given added reason to remind our society that the meaning of life cannot be defined simply by utility, activity, and well-being. Human life includes all kinds of disability and suffering and thus demands solidarity, compassion, and humaneness. When, because of financial restrictions, resources are allocated in a hard and pitiless manner, society's response to its vulnerable old and ill members becomes an even greater sign of its humaneness.

Insofar as the dignity of a person in the concept of the story is not primarily related to a certain degree of cognitive function and ability or to personal efficiency, the differences between mentally and physically "handicapped people" become minor for the question of meaning. But in the concrete care situations, there are indeed important differences. The emphasis of the individual story, in fact, demands arrangements that recognize multifaceted individual problems and resources.

The narrative approach we adopt here emphasizes those models of resource allocation that best support the continuation of the individual life story of the afflicted person. Often outpatient and home health services can provide sufficient support. If long-term care in a nursing home or hospital is necessary, these institutions should promote an atmosphere that respects the individual's dignity and supports the personal resources and relationships of the disabled elderly.

So the concept of meaning, related to individual life stories, has consequences on the micro level of personal relations between the impaired person and the physicians, caregivers, family members, and so on, and on the macro level for all institutions making decisions for resource allocation. On all levels of the social network, this concept signifies more complexity, both of conflicts and of solutions. The aim is a better quality of life for all involved persons and additionally a better and more efficient allocation of resources. Thus, absolutely necessary but not sufficient requirements for implementing a positive meaning of old age hindered by chronic diseases—including the different narratives—are processes of learning on the macro and micro levels by all health care providers. This includes physicians and caregivers, medical and political institutions, engaged peoples in social, political, and educational institutions, and, last but not least, all elderly and disabled persons. It is hoped that as the social negotiations on the allocation of resources continue, an increasing number of elderly people suffering from chronic disease and disorders will become more influential in these conversations.

REFERENCES

1. Bundesministerium für Familie und Senioren (BMFuS), *Erster Altenbericht: Die Lebenssituation älterer Menschen in Deutschland* (First report on the elderly: The life situation of the elderly in Germany) (Bonn: Bundesministerium für Familie und Senioren, 1993), p. 258, Table 2.

2. Klaus Oesterreich, "Altersdemenz, geistige Behinderung, Gebrechlichkeit, körperliche Behinderung" (Dementia in old age, mental handicaps, fragility, physical handicaps), in *Behinderte Menschen im Alter* (Handicapped aged), ed. Norbert Rapp and Werner Strubel (Freiburg: Lambertus, 1992), pp. 132–52. See also B. Bron, "Depression und Suizidalität im Alter" (Depression and tendency to suicide in old age), *Zeitschrift für Gerontologie* 25 (1992): 43–52; H.-J. Möller and A. Rhode, eds., *Psychische Krankheit im Alter* (Mental illness in old age) (New York: Springer, 1993).

3. Gebhard Allert, "Die aktuelle Diskussion um ein neues Pflegeversicherungssystem: politische, soziale, und ethische Aspekte" (The current discussion about a new system of nursing insurance: Political, social, and ethical aspects), *Medizin, Mensch, Gesellschaft* 17 (1992): 47–53. See also E. Rabenstein and U. Schwarzer, "Menschenwürde und Alter: Sozialethische Anmerkungen zur Absicherung des Pflegerisikos" (Human dignity and old age: Social and ethical remarks concerning the prevention of nursing risk), *Zeitschrift für Gerontologie* 25 (1992): 18–24.

4. Dietrich Ritschl, "Altern als Chance und Herausforderung" (Aging as chance and challenge) (paper presented at a congress in Stuttgart, West Germany, 1988). See also Leopold Rosenmayr, *Die späte Freiheit: Das Alter—ein Stück bewusst gelebten Lebens* (The late freedom: Old age—a part of a consciously lived life) (Berlin: Severin and Siedler, 1983).

5. Erik H. Erikson, *Identität und Lebenszyklus* (Identity and life cycle) (Frankfurt: Suhrkamp, 1974), pp. 118–20, 151–52.

6. Anneliese Heigl-Evers and Franz Heigl, "Altern und Psychotherapie: Ein Dialog" (Aging and psychotherapy: A dialogue), *Wege zum Menschen* 44 (1992): 502–12.

7. Dietrich Ritschl and H. Jones, *"Story" als Rohmaterial der Theologie* ("Story" as raw material of theology) (Munich: Kaiser, 1976); Dietrich Ritschl, "Das 'Story'-Konzept in der medizinischen Ethik" (The "story"-concept in medical ethics), *Zeitschrift für Allgemeinmedizin* 58 (1982): 121–26.

8. Juliet M. Corbin and Anselm L. Strauss, *Weiterleben lernen: Chronisch Kranke in der Familie* (Learning to live on: The chronically ill in the family) (Munich: R. Piper, 1993); original edition is *Unending Work and Care* (San Francisco: Jossey-Bass, 1988).

9. Michael Ern, *Wege der Annäherung an die Lebenssituation von älterwerdenden und alten Menschen mit geistiger Behinderung* (Ways of approaching the life situation of aging and elderly people with mental handicaps) (Aachen: Verlag Mainz, 1992), pp. 265–77; see also Gabriele Hermann, "Die Lebensgeschichte—Hilfe für Mitarbeiter" (The life history—aid for coworkers) in Rapp and Strubel, *Behinderte Menschen im Alter*, pp. 211–15.

EVA TOPINKOVÁ

Family Caregiving for the Elderly: Are There Ways to Meet the Need?

The question of filial obligation is an ancient one, and every society and even generation creates its own ideal of the biblical "Honor thy father and mother." Care for old members of the family was always a moral norm in European culture. It came out of the Judeo-Christian moral premise that it is human and moral to care for the old and helpless in the family and in the whole society and that the young and able have responsibility for those who cannot care for themselves. Relationships in the family based on intimacy and mutuality should be fulfilled with mutual honor, love, and affection.

At a general level there is seemingly universal agreement with this premise. This agreement, however, does not make it any easier for us when we seek a concrete application to the individual family. It does not automatically lead us to a universally acceptable model that would tell us how far the duties of children to their parents ought to extend. Nor does it make clear the extent to which our interpretation of those duties is influenced by changing societal conditions and current government policies.

Despite expressed worries that family care is declining and the willingness of family members to give care is decreasing, there is no evidence that this is the case in the contemporary societies of developed countries. Studies from the United States, the United Kingdom, Canada, and Sweden have documented that there is a persistent willingness to give care and that familial caregiving is accepted as a natural human experience.[1] Currently, the majority of care (70 to 80 percent) is provided in the informal sector, mostly by families, with the rest coming from formal paid services provided by professionals.[2]

Yet a willingness to give care represents only the first, though very important, step when family caregivers face the need to provide help. The next two steps are the ability to do so and the knowledge and skills necessary for care. Many families would like to give care if they could, that is, if only the conditions under which they provide care could be more favorable. Many working daughters tell me they would take their parent from the hospital if he or she could walk or if they could rearrange their working schedule, or if . . .

The know-how of home caring is also very important. Virtually all family caregivers are laypeople without any special knowledge of nursing; yet many of the disabled need almost skilled nursing care.

Informal Caregivers and Decision Making

A decision in the family about whether they will be able to manage to care for their frail elderly member is always difficult and often creates a serious moral dilemma. In the decision-making process there are two sets of variables that not only influence the primary decision but predict with high probability how the caregiver will adjust to his or her role and how successfully he or she will go through many months of the unrelieved work of caring. One set of variables is related to the care recipient, the other to the caregiver. External factors outside the family modify further the decision to start and/or continue the caring. These factors include health and social policy, the availability of services and facilities, the way caring is financed, and sociological changes in the society.

Recipient-Related Factors

Geriatric patients are burdened by disability, and that makes them dependent on other people for help and assistance. Of course not all impairments have the same impact on one's dependency level, and not all symptoms are equally difficult for a caregiver to manage. The most socially unacceptable and distressing are those symptoms associated with Alzheimer's disease and other dementias, particularly aggressive, abusive, or disruptive behavior, a disturbance of the day/night cycle, wandering, and permanent double incontinence. Thus the character of the disease and impairment, the level and duration of disability, and the prognosis of the disease are of extreme importance.

One can imagine a family able to care for their acutely ill grandmother who has broken her arm when the caring is short-term and full recovery is expected. The same family would face quite a different situation if, two months later, she suffers a stroke that leaves her bedridden, hemiplegic, and incontinent. In this case caring will be long-standing, recovery improbable, and the prognosis uncertain or poor.

The level of dependency is an important objectively measurable factor and, according to some studies, is inversely related to the amount and extent of care. When an elderly member needs only emotional support, temporary visits and monitoring, and some home help, then most families accept and manage care for many years, even when caregivers work. With further deterioration, when more help and personal assistance is necessary in daily activities such as eating, grooming, toileting, and walking, the caregiver and his or her family have to consider full-time caring, a permanent coresidence situation, giving up a job, and many other things in their personal life. In this situation families seek either paid formal help or permanent placement.

Very often the preparedness of spouse or children to care is influenced substantially by the attitude of the elderly toward the care. Much will depend upon how they perceive their own dependency and whether they can accept the dependent role to be learned and adjusted to. In extreme cases, elderly people refuse care, do not admit the need to be cared for, and prefer their autonomy (better, the feeling that they still are autonomous) and privacy even if it could be dangerous for their health. Many of these are depressed or demented and less than fully competent, and their wishes are influenced by concomitant disease. Others express the view that they would rather die or live in an institution than become dependent on their children or on the mercy of others. When they actually become dependent, however, they not only prefer care by their family but expect it. This ambivalence and uncertainty often prevent them from playing the new role successfully and are a source of stress for both the cared-for and their caregivers.

Caregiver-Related Factors

Among caregiver-related factors age, gender, family composition, socioeconomic status, and quality of familial ties and relationships play an important role. Elderly people turn for help to their closest family members, with the order of preference being spouse, daughter, daughter-in-law, son, and other relatives.[3] As for gender, there are far more women (70–80 percent) than men involved in family caring. Most often the primary caregiver is a spouse, followed closely by daughters. The help of nonrelatives is provided only when a family caregiver is not available. In our sample of 156 dependent elderly, only 5 percent of care was provided by nonrelatives—friends and neighbors—and 0.5 percent of the elderly were cared for by voluntary groups. There is also a clear gender division in the tasks they provide. Sons usually provide financial support and help with heavier household chores, while daughters do the day-to-day work and provide personal care.

The key factors in the decision to provide assistance are the moral and psychological characteristics of the caregiver. In a recent study, Canadian women were asked why they provided care. The factors ranked high (in decreasing order) were love and familial ties, the need to help others, a feeling of duty and obligation, and women's social identity built around caring.[4] As was recently stressed by Ham, these are still positive experiences caregiving provides to both care recipient and caregiver: ". . . Despite the presence of

illness [the cared-for] person can still be enjoyed by the family members. . . .
However, pleasure, joy, love, affection, and an appreciation of excitement,
reminiscence and beauty, and particularly love and affection and many other
life-enhancing qualities are still there to be enjoyed by patient and family
member alike."[5]

Societal Changes and Decreasing Availability of Caregivers

Although care is provided in the context of the individual family, it always
occurs also in the broader societal setting. Many factors outside the family
work in favor of family care, while others make it more difficult. Demographic
changes in all developed countries in the last few decades have increased
substantially the number of elderly people, particularly the oldest old.[6] Because
of the persistently high level of dependency among the elderly, the need for
care increases steadily. It is estimated that 5 to 7 percent of all those sixty-
five and older need institutional placement, and another 20 percent require
care at home. These increasing needs are not matched by an increasing number
of potential caregivers. The number of children between fifty and sixty-four
years relative to dependent elderly parents is dropping, and this trend will
continue in the future (see table 1).[7] In the United Kingdom in 1950, for
example, there were 16.5 elderly over eighty for every 100 women in age-
group fifty to sixty-four. During the next forty years that number rose to 46.6
for every 100 and is expected to rise to 60.2 by 2025. This last figure means
that two-thirds of all women would have a very old parent (currently more
than 50 percent are dependent) to care for.

The demographic situation is not the only factor reducing the relative
availability of caregivers. There are many changes in the social structure of the
family that contribute to this unfavorable development. A declining birthrate, a
decreased number of children in the family, and an increased age of first
pregnancy in many Western European countries and North America together
serve to decrease further the number of potential caregivers. But even those
who are available will be less and less capable of providing care, particularly
because of high and increasing labor force participation by women (table 2),[8]
the geographical distance between the households of children and parents, and
the higher number of divorced, incomplete, or dysfunctional families.

The Stressful Experience of Caregiving

For many primary caregivers and their families, caring for the disabled
old brings a high level of stress. This adverse effect of caregiving affects physical
and mental health, social interaction, and the economic situation of the caring

TABLE 1   Parent Support Ratios between 1950 and 2025 in Selected Countries (Number of Persons 80 Years and Over per 100 Persons Aged 50–64—the Most Probable Caregivers)

Country	Parent Support Ratio			Parent Support Ratio Females		
	1950	1990	2025	1950	1990	2025
Austria	6.6	23.0	30.1	11.7	44.2	60.0
Belgium	8.3	20.6	31.9	15.7	40.0	63.7
Czechoslovakia	6.3	15.6	27.7	11.5	29.3	55.0
Denmark	8.0	24.3	32.2	15.5	47.8	64.7
France	10.1	25.9	31.6	17.9	50.5	62.6
Germany	6.0	19.9	34.3	10.6	39.1	69.1
Hungary	5.3	15.4	33.3	9.6	28.2	66.2
Italy	7.9	17.6	31.8	14.4	33.8	63.4
Sweden	9.3	28.8	38.3	18.0	57.1	76.3
U.K.	9.0	23.7	30.1	16.5	46.6	60.2
U.S.	8.0	21.5	24.6	16.1	41.1	47.8

Source: U.S. Bureau of the Census, *An Aging World II,* International Population Reports p. 25, 92–93 (Washington: U.S. Government Printing Office, 1992) pp. 124, 131–34.

family.[9] Almost two-thirds of those family members who provide care report social problems: disruption of previous social ties inside and outside the family, increasing social distance, loss of friends, no free time or holidays, low social participation, and even isolation. According to a recent American study, about 13 percent of caring daughters had to give up their job altogether and 20 percent experienced conflicting situations at their work place, necessitating rearrangements of their working schedule, reduced working hours, and taking time off without pay.[10] Many working daughters of my own patients experience a very high level of stress because—for economic reasons—they are unable to quit work or even reduce their working hours and at the same time they wish to keep up with their caring duties.

The second most frequently reported negative consequence is a deterioration of the health of the caregiver; the older the caregiver, the greater the health problems. Women in general complain about this more than males. As many as 30 percent of children caring for older parents experience a decline in physical health.[11] They suffer from sleeplessness, back pain, and physical exhaustion. Long-standing family care demands enormous commitments and adaptations that cause emotional and psychological problems. Many caregivers also report guilt feelings, helplessness, frustration, anger, aggression, substance abuse, and even overt mental-health deterioration with symptomatic anxiety or depression. To make matters worse, they feel unhappy and guilty about

TABLE 2 Labor Force Participation of Women of Different Ages in 1980s in Selected Countries

	Percent of Working Women in a Given Age-Group			
Country	*50–54*	*55–59*	*60–64*	*65+*
Austria	51.6	24.6	5.7	0.9
Belgium	30.7	17.3	5.7	1.0
Czechoslovakia	79.9	40.8	21.5	6.5
Denmark	49.5	39.8	24.9	4.6
France	54.1	41.4	18.0	2.1
Germany (West)	53.7	41.1	11.1	1.8
Hungary	67.4	18.8	8.7	2.9
Italy	34.1	20.2	9.8	2.2
Sweden	83.1	72.5	45.6	3.1
U.K.	63.5	51.5	18.8	2.7
U.S.	59.2	50.2	34.2	7.9

Source: U.S. Bureau of the Census, *An Aging World II,* International Population Reports p. 25, 92–93 (Washington: U.S. Government Printing Office, 1992) pp. 124, 131–34.

their conflicting feelings toward their parents. Those feelings distort the previously healthy mutual ties of affection, converting them to permanent distress. Often we can detect the burnout syndrome, overt or hidden signs of abusive behavior, or neglect of the elder.

The last but not least important problem is the financial cost of caring. These costs are either direct expenses (such as for medication, diet or housing rearrangements, and outside help) or indirect expenses caused by lost income when a caregiver gives up a paid job.

The negative consequences of caring among a substantial proportion of caregivers make them a group at risk. They need help and support from professionals but also from other family members and society at large. This so-called care for caregivers is sometimes more important than the care for the disabled ones. It helps to explain the large amount of literature focusing on caregiver stress, on its measurement, and on possible intervention to buffer or mitigate the ill effects of caregiving.[12] But what are the effective and feasible intervention strategies, and which policy would best respond to caregiver needs?

Care for Caregivers: Policy Implications

All countries facing long-term-care problems are adopting policies that are centered on relieving part of the caregiving burden (table 3). The reason for this intervention is also economic. It is expected that less burdened caregivers will not only feel better and probably care better; they will be able to continue caring for their elderly at home for a longer period of time. Expensive institutional placement will be reduced or at least postponed, and public money thus saved.

The first step in relieving a caregiver's stress is its identification and measurement. The key role of the primary-care family practitioner and the community nurse in this assessment has been stressed by the American Medical Association:

> [There is] the key linkage role of the primary care physician who recognizes that caregivers and patients form interdependent units, and [who] affirm a care partnership between the physician and caregiver. . . . [He] conducts periodic assessments of the caregiver as well as the patient, uses a comprehensive home-based approach to care and services, provides training to caregivers, particularly in managing difficult behavior, validates the role of caregiver, and acts as case manager.[13]

There are still weak incentives and a lack of proper education, however, for primary-care physicians to do all of these things, even if the beneficial effects have been proven. Among other more or less still experimental methods of social support are individual counseling and education and group intervention. Toseland et al. and Mittelman et al. found that both professional and peer counseling improved the psychological functioning and well-being of caregivers and reduced the level of the overall strain.[14] The most effective activities were social interaction conducted with friends and family members outside the family, just for fun, pleasure, and recreation.[15] Involvement in self-help support groups also could be helpful, but this form of help is more important in countries where the voluntary sector has worked for decades and where interest groups are involved in political life. The countries of Southern and Eastern Europe are only slowly discovering such benefits.

One of the controversial problems is the utilization of community and home care services by caring families. These services were originally developed for people who were childless or lived alone or whose children did not care. Now they are used more and more also by caregivers who are heavily burdened or who work and cannot provide care during the usual working hours. But there is a fear that utilization of services might negatively influence the willingness of caregivers to continue caring. Some recent findings from the United States and Europe, however, showed that nowhere has home care substituted for family caring. On the contrary, services such as housekeeping, meals-on-wheels, personal-care services, home sitting, or professional health care (home

TABLE 3   Ill Effects of Caring, and Interventions Relieving Caregiver's Burden

Area	Danger	Intervention
Physical	Ill health, psychosomatic diseases	Periodic health checkups by general practitioner, rehabilitation aids, professional assistance, day and respite care
Psychological	Emotional stress	Individual and group counseling
Emotional	Mental-health problems, anxiety, depression, low self-esteem, loss of control	Psychotherapy, appreciation and emotional support, respite care
Social	Social isolation, loneliness, restriction of social activities	Social-support network, self-help groups, social-worker help, home sitting, respite care
Financial	Poverty	Home care allowance, care leave payment

occupational therapy, speech therapy) can substantially help those families who otherwise would not be able to cope with elderly needs.[16] Although these services seem to be widely available, their utilization is still low, particularly among caregivers who are old, less educated, and depressed.[17]

In the last decade there has been more research work on experimental respite care programs. Respite care usually takes the form of temporary (time-limited) admissions to an institution, either to the acute- or long-term-care wards of a hospital or to nursing or residential homes. This intervention aims to help the family to relieve the stress of unremitting care.[18] Although respite care can alleviate the burden and level of subjective stress of the caregiver, it does not prevent permanent institutionalization. Moreover, there are some dangers in this intervention for frail, dependent elderly. New faces, a hospital-like regime, often more aggressive treatment, and the change from a known home environment increase the risk for the patient, particularly those with dementia. The adverse events connected with hospitalization of the old are delirium (10–15 percent), trauma (10 percent), institution-acquired infection, and iatrogenic adverse-effect drug reaction (8 percent each). Even if a recent study of Chang et al. did not report increased risk of mortality or iatrogenesis,[19] my own experience with respite care would recommend a more cautious approach. The most suitable forms of respite are day care centers, providing care during the day and enabling the patient to stay home overnight.

When it is no longer possible for the elderly patient to be cared for at home, the family confronts a difficult and painful decision, whether and where to place their old parent or grandparent. The risk of institutionalization is high in cases of heavy dependence on basic personal care, of disruptive behavior, and of a perceived inadequacy of the home services. Even more important are the subjective feelings of the caregiver, who might not be able to cope even with lower levels of stress. The third important factor is the acceptance of an institutional alternative and the availability of a proper institution at the right time. Individual countries differ in the types and relative number of institutions. In most countries, however, the societal attitude toward long-term-care institutions is more or less negative. They are looked upon as the last resort, where those who have been abandoned by their family members live their last, most disabled years of life. Though much has changed in the quality of care and in the quality of life of the institutionalized, the negative image of those institutions still persists among old people and their caregivers. Placement often reminds the family of the finality of the life of the old and the irreversibility and failure of the caregiver's role. The old member often remains passive ("They put me into the old people's home"), and the whole responsibility lies on the shoulder of the caregiver. It is often a source of further stress and guilt.

One of the prevailing myths is that the permanent placement of the dependent elderly member into an institution relieves all of the stress and necessity of caring. But our parents remain still our parents, waiting for our love and affection even if they are in the institution, and probably even more so. Recent American studies have confirmed that children and spouses continue caring for their institutionalized elderly, and they spend a great deal of time doing so.[20]

All of the above-mentioned interventions are meant to relieve physical and emotional strain. There are, however, other measures that can help families to continue caregiving. Direct financial support to a care recipient or to his or her caregiver, or different forms of care allowances, or care leaves or services provided free of charge are examples of possible economic support. They not only help directly but, importantly, are a way of implementing into social policy a societal appreciation and reward for caring families. The task for future health and social policy is to create conditions in which the family can share responsibility with the governmental and formal sector.

Family caregiving has an irreplaceable role in caring for the dependent old. Caregiving, however, should be an act of free choice and personal commitment of both the caregiver and the care recipient, not their duty in a situation in which outside help and alternative forms of care are not available. Only then can the dependent elderly preserve their dignity and freedom and find, in the family, the place where they belong.

REFERENCES

1. J. Finch and J. Mason, "Filial Obligations and Kin Support for Elderly People," *Aging and Society* 10 (1990): 151–75; N. Guberman, P. Maheu, and C. Maillé "Women as Family Caregivers: Why Do They Care?" *Gerontologist* 32, no. 5 (1992): 607–17; S. L. Tennstedt, S. L. Crawford, and J. B. McKinley, "Is Family on the Decline? A Longitudinal Investigation of the Substitution of Formal Long-Term Care Services for Informal Care," *Milbank Memorial Fund Quarterly* 71, no. 4 (1993): 601–24; N. Carlsson-Agren, S. Berg, C. G. Wenestam, "The Oldest Old and Their Children: How Strong Are the Relationships?" *Aging* (Milano) 4, no. 4 (1992): 293–300: C. Wolfson et al., "Adult Children's Perceptions of Their Responsibility to Provide Care for Dependent Elderly Parents," *Gerontologist* 33, no. 3 (1993): 315–23; E. Topinková, "What Do Children Owe Their Old Dependent Elderly? Moral Dilemmas of Family Care," in *Proceedings of the World Pro-Life Conference*, ed. J. Glasa and M. Mikolášik (forthcoming).

2. G. Dooghe, "Informal Caregivers of Elderly People: A European Review," *Ageing and Society* 12 (1992): 369–80.

3 Ibid.

4. Guberman et al., "Women as Family Caregivers."

5. R. J. Ham, "Alzheimer's Disease and the Family: A Challenge of the New Millennium," *Advances in Experimental Medicine and Biology* 282 (1990): 3–20.

6. U.S. Bureau of the Census, *An Aging World II*, International Population Reports P25, 92–3, (Washington: U.S. Government Printing Office, 1992), pp. 124, 13–34.

7. Ibid.

8. Ibid.

9. Dooghe, "Informal Caregivers of Elderly People"; B. Hirshorn, "Family Caregiving as an Intergenerational Transfer," in *Health, Illness, and Disability in Later Life: Practice Issues and Interventions*, ed. R. F. Young and E. A. Olson (London: Sage, 1991).

10. E. M. Brody et al., "Work Status and Parent Care: A Comparison of Four Groups of Women," *Gerontologist* 27, no. 2 (1987): 201–8.

11. Dooghe, "Informal Caregivers of Elderly People."

12. E. A. Mohide et al, "A Randomized Trial of Family Caregiver Support in the Home Management of Dementia," *Journal of the American Geriatric Society* 38, no. 4 (1990): 446–54; Council on Scientific Affairs, American Medical Association, "Physicians and Family Caregivers: A Model for Partnership," *JAMA* 269, no. 10 (1993): 1282–84; E. H. Thompson et al., "Social Support and Caregiving Burden in Family Caregivers of Frail Elders," *Journal of Gerontology* 48, no. 5 (1993): S245–S254.

13. Council on Scientific Affairs, "Physicians and Family Caregivers."

14. R. W. Toseland et al., "Comparative Effectiveness of Individual and Group Intervention to Support Family Caregivers," *Social Work* 35, no. 3 (1990): 209–17; M. S. Mittelman et al., "An Intervention That Delays Institutionalization of Alzheimer's Disease Patients: Treatment of Spouse Caregivers," *Gerontologist* 33, no. 6 (1993): 730–40.

15. Thompson et al., "Social Support."

16. M. A. Neary, "Community Services in the 1990s: Are They Meeting the Needs of Caregivers?" *Journal of Community Health Nursing* 19, no. 2 (1993): 105–11.

17. C. Collins et al., "Knowledge and Use of Community Services among Family Caregivers of Alzheimer's Disease Patients," *Archives of Psychiatric Nursing* 5, no. 2 (1991): 84–90.

18. J. P. Larkin and B. M. Hopcroft, "In-Hospital Respite as a Moderator of Caregiver Stress," *Health and Social Work* 19, no. 2 (1993): 132–38.

19. J. I. Chang et al., "Patient Outcomes in Hospital-Based Respite: A Study of Potential Risks and Benefits," *Journal of the American Board of Family Practitioners* 5, no. 5 (1992): 475–81.

20. S. King et al., "Institutionalization of an Elderly Family Member: Reaction of Spouse and Nonspouse Caregivers," *Archives of Psychiatric Nursing* 5, no. 6 (1991): 323–30; G. J. Stevens, R. A. Walsh, and B. A. Baldwin, "Family Caregivers of Institutionalized and Noninstitutionalized Elderly Individuals," *Nursing Clinics of North America* 28, no. 2 (1993): 349–62; M. S. Moss et al., "Time Use of Caregivers of Impaired Elders before and after Institutionalization," *Journal of Gerontology* 48, no. 3 (1993): S102–S111.

SARAH-VAUGHAN BRAKMAN

Adult Daughter Caregivers: Philosophical Analysis and Implications for Health Care Policy

As part of the discussion on resource allocation for the aged, it is crucial to ask not only who the family caregivers are and whether they need assistance but also how the conceptual underpinning of obligations of caregiving can contribute to a more just allocation. This chapter examines only one type of family caregiving, that of adult children to parents. It focuses particularly on the experience of adult daughters as caregivers. A conceptual analysis of the basis of filial obligations is provided in an attempt to deal with some of the dilemmas experienced by these caregivers.

Adult Daughters and the Care of the Aged

The stereotype that the elderly in the United States are abandoned by their families and "warehoused" in nursing homes is a myth.[1] Only 5 percent of the elderly in the United States are institutionalized. Nine in ten of the disabled elderly not in nursing homes receive unpaid care from relatives and friends. Up to seven million Americans are unpaid caregivers to the elderly, and most are women.[2] Adult daughters and daughters-in-law are the principal helpers of older people who care for disabled spouses, and they are the primary caregivers to the more than nine million widowed older people who are dependent.[3] In the United States, the current average caregiver to the elderly is forty-five years old, female, and married. Among children who are primary caregivers, daughters outnumber sons three to one.[4]

A number of demographic changes have increased the strain on informal caregiving for women in particular. Americans eighty-five and older, the group most in need of long-term care, are the fastest growing segment of the population, but since the baby boomers have created a baby bust by having fewer children, the ranks of future caregivers will be depleted. Furthermore, unlike their mothers, greater numbers of women will enter the work force

TABLE 1   Women and Filial Obligation

Tradition	Filial Obligation
Greek	Helps with duties of husband; only father esteemed
Imperial Chinese	After marriage, obligation to parents replaced by obligation to in-laws; bond to mother-in-law more important than marital bond
Judaic	Obligation to one's own parents remains, with addition of helping the husband; mother held in equal esteem with father
Christian	Father and mother held in equal honor and love
Islamic	Mother has elevated status over father

and stay there. The need for affordable, quality elder and child care will increase.[5]

These observations mean that there are more elderly and fewer adult children to care for them and that unlike the past, parent care is often a time-extended process that lasts for years, with women in particular shouldering heavy, often unbearable burdens.

Selected Background of Gender-Specific Filial Caregiving

The current predominance of adult daughters and daughters-in-law as caregivers is rooted in philosophical, sociological, cultural, and religious traditions. The findings of a select survey on filial obligations and women as viewed by influential homogenous cultural and religious traditions are presented in table 1.[6]

The focus of filial obligations in the written historical texts is on what sons owe to their parents, with emphasis on what sons owe to fathers. In the patriarchal traditions listed in the table, women in marriage are necessary helpers to husbands fulfilling their filial obligations. For example, the Chinese and the Jewish traditions both hold this view. In the traditional Chinese culture, daughters are married into the family of their husband. At the same time, obligations of care to their parents cease. They are obligated to their husband and to their husband's parents. Unfilial conduct to a husband's parents was one of the seven reasons that a man could divorce his wife. But respecting the mourning time (three years) for either or both of her in-laws was one of the three sanctions that protected a woman from divorce by her husband. Such behavior in prerevolutionary China was consider the "the highest act of filial duty."[7] In the classic work "The Twenty-Four Examples of Filial Piety," a woman's care of parents is only mentioned in reference to her in-laws. In the eleventh example, a woman walked a great distance every day to get from a river the water that her mother-in-law loved to drink. It is said that the son's wife "fulfilled her mother-in-law's commands without the least reluctance."[8] This devotion was upheld as a standard for daughters-in-law to follow.

According to the tenets of the Jewish tradition, daughters are required to obey and respect parents, but after their marriage, they are responsible primarily to their husbands.[9] Wives assume with their husbands the obligations to take care of his parents. The Mishnah states that "all obligations of the father upon the son, both men and women are bound."[10] One of the Rabbis says:

> All precepts concerning a father, which are incumbent upon son to perform for his father, both men and women are bound thereby. We have (thus) learnt here what our Rabbis taught: (Ye shall fear every man his father, and his mother): "man," I know it only of man; how do I know it of woman? When it is said, "Ye shall fear," two are mentioned. If so, why state *man*? A man possesses the means to fulfil this, but woman has no means of fulfilling this, because she is under the authority of others. R. Idi B. Abin said in Rab's name: If she is divorced, both are equal.[11]

This is conceptually different from the Chinese obligations to parents-in-law because the Chinese owe these obligations directly to the spouse's parents after marriage. The Jewish tradition holds that a wife is helping her husband by honoring his parents, rather than, as Gerald Blidstein notes, reflecting "a new 'filial' bond linking the extended family."[12] In what women owe their own parents after marriage, the comparison between Chinese and Judaic views is even more interesting: After marriage for the Chinese, obligations toward a woman's parents are, theoretically, negated. The Jewish position, however, holds that such obligations still exist theoretically, but the tradition recognizes the practical difficulty of fulfilling these after marriage.

Writings from Revolutionary American women show that filial duty was gender specific, with sons expected to provide financial contributions and daughters to provide the hands-on care and nurture of aged parents. Women perceived their responsibility as both appropriate and necessary within the prescribed limits of a woman's sphere. Caregiving was appropriate to their training and to peculiarly "feminine" characteristics. Women felt obligated to repay parents (usually mothers) for the care of nurturing provided in childhood.[13]

Present-day data on the effects of women's changing roles on attitudes toward responsibility for care of elderly adults reflect significant generational differences about the sharing of parent care and household tasks by men and women. In a study of three generations of women by Elaine Brody, the women in each generation were in favor of such sharing, though the youngest generation was most in favor of egalitarian gender roles.[14] Interestingly, Brody reports, "at the same time [the youngest generation] expected to work much longer than their mothers and grandmothers had expected to work when *they* were young women even though the granddaughters expected to marry and to have as many children as their mothers and grandmothers. In short, they expect to do it all."[15] What leads this youngest generation to believe they can "do it all?" Is it that they receive more sharing from males than their foremothers, or is it that even though women's roles have changed, societal expectations, and the expectations of women caregivers themselves, have not changed? Women, not men, are expected to give up their job if elder caregiving is needed. Even if they do not stop working, women who work still spend the same amount of time in elder care.[16] When men do share the caregiving, the tasks are still considered to be traditionally gender specific. Men usually help with transportation, home repairs, and financial management rather than with personal care. It is this personal care, though, that is more intensive and enduring.

Caregiving Dilemmas for Adult Daughters

In addition to bearing the greatest proportion of the caregiving burden, adult daughters have to balance the obligations of elder caregiving with other special obligations, such as those to their young children, to their spouses, to their employers, and to themselves. At least 1.8 million women are simultaneously caring for children and coping with elder care responsibilities. Over half of these women are also in the paid labor force. One in five women has a parent living in her home.[17] "With a longer life expectancy and no public health care coverage of chronic illness, many women can expect to spend their 'golden years' drained of their income from a caregiving experience." Not only do these women lose their income and security; they often forfeit their health. Many suffer from what has become known as "caregiver's syndrome." Caregiver's syndrome is "developed from years of physical strain in the care of parents and then spouses. Lifting and turning a disabled adult can result in bursitis, can damage the spine and lower back, and can quicken the advance of osteoporosis. Repetitive, heavy lifting can increase even younger caregivers' chances of developing arthritis."[18] Merely two hundred of the six million employers in the United States offer any assistance with elder care. Half of these companies only provide long-term-care insurance.[19]

Few options exist for families with elder care responsibilities. Nursing homes are a question of cost, space, and quality. Discrimination against the poor is rampant in the competition for limited nursing home beds. Adult day care centers exist nationwide, but there are long waiting lists to get into these programs which can cost up to thirty dollars a day or more.[20]

Many women reach the limit of their endurance trying to balance the needs of an elder parent with those of the rest of the family in an effort to avoid nursing home placement. When elder parents do take up residence in a nursing home, this is often experienced by the child and the elder as a moral, emotional, and physical failure. Failure is also experienced when daughter caregivers must turn to formal care services for assistance. This failure seems to say, "You (the parent) loved me and never abandoned me, but I couldn't handle it for you." Siblings of primary caregivers feel guilt as well, with female siblings experiencing more guilt than their brothers.[21] The dilemma for women is that no matter how much they do, it is never enough to repay their parents or to meet all the needs of the parents, and that is what daughters especially believe they ought to do for elder parents.

Conceptual Analysis

Adult daughter caregivers implicitly appeal to reciprocity as the basis of filial obligations. Failure to provide the same quality, quantity, and intensity of care as their parents provided to them as young children is viewed as a moral failure. Failure to put obligations to parents as the first priority, just as parents put obligations to their young children as the first priority, is considered a moral failure on the part of adult children, especially daughters, who are believed and expected to be more "natural" caregivers than sons. Social norms and ethnic religious and cultural values are powerful reinforcements for such expectations.

An example of the belief that filial responsibilities are grounded in a notion of reciprocity is found in Blackstone's *Commentaries on the Laws of England*:

> The duties of children to their parents arise from a principle of natural justice and retribution. For to those who gave us existence we naturally owe subjection and obedience during our minority, and honor and reverence ever after; they who protected the weakness of our infancy are entitled to our protection in the infirmity of their age; they who by sustenance and education have enabled their offspring to prosper ought in return to be supported by that offspring in case they stand in need of assistance.[22]

Blackstone believed children ought to return to parents the same type of benefits that the parents provided to the children when the parents likewise become in need.

There are, however, many problems with viewing reciprocity as the philosophical basis of filial obligations. One of the most important considerations of reciprocity-based filial obligations is that it is impossible to repay parents. What would count as repayment for being given life or for all that was provided during child rearing? The question remains without answer. Furthermore, any repayment would always be in response to what the parents did, and hence, as Kant says, one could never repay the spontaneous benevolence of another who was the first to give.[23] Since "ought" implies "can," it is not possible to have obligations that have no logical possibility of being able to be met. For this reason, reciprocity cannot be the conceptual basis of filial obligations, yet it is the basis to which adult daughters at least implicitly appeal. Seeing that conceptually it does not work might account for, and make some sense of, the frustration and confusion that adult daughters have when they try to meet so-called reciprocity-based filial obligations.

Furthermore, a reciprocity account of filial obligations implies that when debts are repaid, the morally significant relationship is over and one is "free" of obligations. If filial obligations were solely obligations of reciprocity, what would be the status of the parent–adult child relationship before the obligation of reciprocity? This question is meaningless, since the child—and hence the possibility of any relationship—did not exist before the existence of the obligation. For adoptive parents, the status of the original relationship was that of strangers. Can we meaningfully say that after reciprocity-based obligations are fulfilled, the child owes parents no more than what strangers owe one another? The answer is clearly "no." There will always be a unique connection to one's parents. As Daniel Callahan states, "The emotional and biological bond between parent and child gives the relationship a permanent and central place in our lives, quite apart from whether that relationship turns out well or poorly."[24]

The moral basis of filial obligation is better understood as an obligation of gratitude for all the parent has done for the child. This account is different from reciprocity, for it is not characterized by repayment (though there may be compensation for a sacrifice). Gratitude is a response of appreciation and goodwill, on the part of the adult child, directed toward the benevolence of the parent for providing the important and unique benefits needed in childhood. The conditions necessary for gratitude to be due parents include the facts that parents provided benefits of life and/or caregiving to their children voluntarily, benevolently, and primarily for the sake of the child alone and that the benefits provided were considered socially valuable. If these conditions obtain, then children have an obligation to cultivate attitudes of gratitude and goodwill and to do those acts which demonstrate the possession of such attitudes. I argue elsewhere for why it is these particular conditions which are necessary for gratitude to be due and for why gratitude is the moral foundation of filial obligation.[25]

Gratitude obligations are neither absolute, unlimited, nor inherently overriding. "That the moral claim made upon them [caregivers] may seem a justifiable one in many respects does not mean that it will be endurable; that it is endurable does not mean that it is justifiable."[26] Gratitude duties may also be viewed as prima facie obligations, meaning obligations that must be met, provided there exists no equally compelling obligation that must also be met. Seen in this way, the rightness of acts can only be judged by determining, for an agent in a certain circumstance, which act has the "greatest balance of prima facie rightness ... over prima facie wrongness."[27] Gratitude seems to lack the specificity that enables one to decide this balance—a problem that may rightly reflect the complexity and ambiguity of the subject matter of filial responsibilities. It is not unusual to see four generations in a family, with a forty-five-year-old caring for young children, a seventy-year-old mother, and a ninety-year-old grandmother. How does the gratitude account aid this person in determining his or her duties? In one instance of competing obligations, however, it is perhaps possible to adjudicate the balance. When filial obligations and obligations to young children are both present and in direct conflict, then because obligations are generally considered to be forward flowing, obligations to the younger generations at least to some extent override filial duties.[28]

The gratitude account perhaps can ease some of the dilemmas of adult daughters by showing: (1) obligations are present for all adult children—sons and daughters—who received relevant benefits from parents and while one child may voluntarily assume the role of primary caregiver, other children of the parent ought to fulfill filial obligations of gratitude through other means; (2) sometimes obligations to parents do not exist, as in the case of parents who were neglectful of their parental obligations or who abused their children; and (3) even when filial obligations of caregiving exist, sometimes these obligations legitimately cannot be met because of the existence of competing special obligations or must be met in limited ways that still demonstrate the attitudes of appreciation and goodwill.

Implications for Health Care Policy

Family caregivers are predominately female because the role is viewed as part of the feminine sphere, part of the activities and skills associated with women as mothers. "Caring," meaning both compassion and doing for others, however, is not uniquely feminine. As shown by the experience of adult daughter caregivers, women especially and families in general cannot meet all of the needs of the elderly, nor should they be required to do so. Most adult children have some level of gratitude obligation that requires them to help with the care of their parents. But as seen here, these obligations are neither unlimited nor absolute. How can this help shape public policy in the United States on family care of the elderly?

First, there is a need to reach society and caregivers with the message that filial obligations of caregiving must be met by all adult children who have such responsibilities and not by daughters as a matter of default. Disseminating this message will include reshaping societal expectations regarding women, as well as continued discussion of the implications of obligations and gratitude. Second, in the national and international dialogue on intergenerational justice, it is important to realize that special obligations of gratitude within families do exist. This does not mean that public policy should engage in the enforcement of such obligations. Such action would most probably be counterproductive to promoting the cultivation of attitudes of gratitude in adult children. Third, the state should, nevertheless, be actively supportive of families trying to meet filial obligations of gratitude. Such support can take the form of financial subsidies for family caregivers who cannot afford to quit working to care for an elderly parent. The Family and Medical Leave Act, recently enacted in the United States, provides job protection for caregivers of children, parents, and spouses, but the leave is without pay and for a limited time. Health care reform must include funding for long-term care services such as home health care, respite care, and adult day care services. Third, formal-care and home care services must be radically improved so people will not feel they are abandoning their elders when reliance on such services is appropriate or necessary. This includes training and screening for nursing home aides and employees as well as federally funded adult day care centers. Measures like these would allow many adult children to meet their gratitude obligations to parents while balancing equally important special obligations to other family members and themselves. Filial obligations of caregiving exist, and most people want to care for their parents, whether obligations exist or not. Public policy should make it easier for individuals to do so, rather than force some citizens to bear all of the burdens.

REFERENCES

1. Drew Christiansen, "Ethical Guidelines for Assisting the Elderly," *America* 156, no. 4 (1987): 72–75, at 72. See also Berta G. Simos, "Relations of Adults with Aging Parents," *Gerontologist* 10, no. 2 (1970): 135–39; and *Failing America's Caregivers: A Status Report on Women Who Care* (Older Women's League, May 1989), p. 3.

2. *Failing America's Caregivers*, p. 2.

3. Elaine M. Brody, "Filial Care of the Elderly and Changing Roles of Women (and Men)," *Journal of Geriatric Psychiatry* 19, no. 2 (1986): 175–201, at 177–78.

4. *Failing America's Caregivers*, p. 3.

5. Ibid., pp. 4–5.

6. Sarah-Vaughan Brakman, "A Philosophical Analysis of Filial Obligations" (Ph.D. diss., Rice University, 1994), pp. 25–129.

7. G. Jamieson, *Chinese Family and Commercial Law* (Hong Kong: Vetch and Lee, 1970), pp. 41, 53.

8. *The Book of Filial Duty*, trans. Ivan Chen (London: John Murray, 1908), p. 45.

9. *Encyclopedia of Religion and Ethics*, 1913 ed., s.v. "family."

10. *The Babylonian Talmud*, trans. I. Epstein (London: Soncino Press, 1935), Kiddush 29a.

11. Ibid., Kiddush 30b.

12. *Mo'ed katon* 206, cited in Gerald Blidstein, *Honor Thy Father and Mother: Filial Responsibility in Jewish Law and Ethics* (New York: Ktav, 1975), p. 99.

13. Terri Premo, " 'A Blessing to Our Declining Years': Feminine Response to Filial Duty in the New Republic," *International Journal of Aging and Human Development* 20, no. 1 (1984–85): 69–74, at 73.

14. Brody, "Filial Care of the Elderly," p. 179; Elaine M. Brody et al., "Women's Changing Roles and Help to Elderly Parents: Attitudes of Three Generations of Women," *Journal of Gerontology* 38, no. 5 (1983): 597–607.

15. Ibid., p. 180.

16. Ibid., p. 4.

17. Ibid., p. 3.

18. Ibid., p. 8.

19. Ibid., p. 9.

20. Ibid., p. 6.

21. Brody, "Filial Care of the Elderly," p. 185.

22. William Blackstone, *Commentaries on the Laws of England* (Philadelphia: J. B. Lippincott, 1856), vol. 1, bk. 1, chap. 16, sec. 1, cited in Jeffrey Blustein, *Parents and Children: The Ethics of the Family* (New York: Oxford University Press, 1982), p. 181.

23. Immanuel Kant, *The Metaphysics of Morals*, trans. Mary Gregor (Cambridge: Cambridge University Press, 1991), p. 249.

24. Daniel Callahan, "What Do Children Owe Elderly Parents?" *Hastings Center Report* 15, no. 2 (1985): 32–37, at 35.

25. Sarah-Vaughan Brakman, "Filial Responsibility and Long-Term Care Decision Making," in *Long-Term Care Decisions: Ethical and Conceptual Dimensions*, ed. Laurence B. McCullough and Nancy L. Wilson (Baltimore: Johns Hopkins University Press), 1995.

26. Daniel Callahan, "Families as Caregivers: The Limits of Morality, " *Archives of Physical Medicine Rehabilitation* 69 (May 1988): 323–28, at 323.

27. D. W. Ross, *The Right and the Good* (Oxford: Clarendon Press, 1930), pp. 41–42.

28. Henry Sidgwick, *The Methods of Ethics* (Chicago: University of Chicago Press, 1962).

Parts of this article were previously published in Sarah-Vaughan Brakman, "Adult Daughter Caregivers" *Hastings Center Report* 24, no. 5 (1994): 26–28, and Sarah-Vaughan Brakman, "Filial Responsibility and Long-Term Care Decision Making" in *Long-Term Care Decisions: Ethical and Conceptual Dimensions*, eds. Laurence B. McCullogh and Nancy L. Wilson (Baltimore: Johns Hopkins University Press), 1995.

BELA BLASSZAUER

Institutional Care of the Elderly: Lessons from Hungary

There is no reason to doubt that a society can indeed very well be judged on the basis of how it takes care of its elderly. By assuring high-quality care, whether by providing it directly in public institutions or by supporting private caregivers, society could demonstrate its appreciation to a whole generation. High-quality care is an ethical concern in at least two senses: providing good care for the elderly is itself an ethical obligation; and care must be provided in an ethical manner, that is, the human dimensions of care ought to take the central place.

Both the elderly themselves and younger generations can benefit when the old are assured good care. A pleasant, comfortable old age, either in an institution or at home, would show the young and middle-aged generations that they have ample time left in life to achieve certain desires and to realize their human potentials. It would teach that life is not meaningless and devoid of quality beyond the age of retirement, that the young and middle-aged need not be greedy and egotistical, rushing to acquire all that they can before life inevitably ends at retirement.

Only a good old age can give real meaning to the spectacular extension of the life span that medicine now makes possible. And only a good old age can help restore a more balanced model for younger generations. Given the tremendous technical progress with which a ten-year-old is more acquainted than a seventy-year-old, it might be true today that the old cannot claim much special knowledge that the younger ones would seek to learn from them. Only a good old age can help restore respect for the experiential wisdom that can be passed on from generation to generation.

Hans-Georg Gadamer, the ninety-three-year-old German philosopher, said in an interview, "I am a living anachronism, because I don't belong to this world any more, but I am still here."[1] Surveys carried out among the elderly show the same or a similar view. We need a culture of old age if we want generations to live in harmony and if we want the elderly to enjoy a certain quality of life, including an acceptable degree of self-esteem and meaningful human relationships. Gadamer refers to social homes or homes for the aged as perfect schools for rapid aging. Some Hungarian health administrators call them "the places for collective dying"; others refer to them as "houses for the poor or forgotten people." In Hungary no humanistic care for the elderly has developed yet that would secure old age against existential fear and anxiety.

Aging in Hungary

In Hungary old age—according to the general view of the society—begins at the time of retirement, even if there are no visible signs of biological or bodily deterioration. At present the retirement age is sixty for men and fifty-five for women. The number of retired people has grown to over two and a half million, from 20.7 percent to almost 22 percent in recent years. Some forty-three thousand people receive regular social aid, while emergency help is given to over half a million people annually. Yet as the number of people who need places in social homes grows, the number of places is decreasing. And as Laszlo Vertes, the general secretary of the Hungarian Gerontological Society noted: "The number of personnel is inadequate, . . . though the care of the elderly is three-dimensional: psychic, bodily, and social. The old justly feel that they don't deserve such lousy treatment from society after so many decades of work."[2]

Among the institutions providing care for the elderly in Hungary are social homes, day care centers, home care, and apartments for retired people. Principally there are four types of social homes: for the elderly, for the mentally ill, for alcoholics, and for others. Often, however, the population of these homes is very heterogeneous, and the mixing of relatively healthy people with the retarded, the mentally ill, alcoholics, and young and old homeless individuals creates a number of problems. According to 1992 figures from Hungary's Central Statistics Office, there were 25,279 places in social homes, with 11,385 employees. Of these places, 21,989 belonged to local government, 2,122 to churches, 345 to private enterprise, 68 to foundations, 59 to societies, and 331 to others.

Arguably, security at Los Alamos during the Manhattan Project was not as strict as at some of our social homes. Although our research on the ethical aspects of institutional care is financially supported by the Hungarian National Research Fund, my colleagues had great difficulties interviewing residents. In many places it was simply not allowed; in others, the interviewer was allowed to go into only those rooms assigned to her by the institution's administrators. At times, an administration representative accompanied the interviewer every-where, so that residents were not able to speak candidly. Nevertheless, at a few institutions enough information could be collected to draw a general picture of the prevailing morals of institutional care.

Publicly funded "social homes" or "welfare homes," as they are known in Hungary, are intended to be residential facilities for those who are not seriously ill but who require assistance with daily activities and cannot be adequately cared for through day care centers or daytime home care. These homes are not designed to provide skilled care and supervision around the clock. Beyond being called upon to give a level of care they are not really equipped to provide, social homes evolved out of the older system of "poor houses" and so are much stigmatized.

Most residents of social homes have only an elementary-school education. They are people who have gone through world wars, revolution, foreign occupation, mass urbanization and industrialization, and many personal tragedies. Most of those who receive care in an institution are men, since in Hungary divorce laws favor women, and men may be left without a roof over their heads. In addition, some women and men have been involuntarily committed to social homes.

Residents often become second-class citizens who must defer to staff and whose lives are regimented by the needs of the institution. Thus at one social home with 220 elderly residents, the strict daily routine of personal care (bathing, dressing, medications, etc.), meals, and limited social activities begins with awakening at 5:00 AM in a schedule that runs through "lights out" at 8:00 PM. Residents must get permission to leave the home and must return before gates are locked in the evening. Those whose behavior disrupts the order of the home face possible disciplinary action by its social committee.[3]

Because of the lingering stigma of these former "poor houses," the more well-to-do place their relatives in hospitals and sanatoria, since it is embarrassing to put one's parents in the social homes. In Hungary, there is no institutional form to accommodate the very sick and immobile people who need continuous care. Hospital beds can be utilized for this purpose, though geriatric wards are quite rare. In general, hospital beds and such wards should be reserved for those who have a good chance for continuous improvement in their state of health, if not a full recovery. In the town of Pécs, for example, there is a geriatric hospital ward where university clinics and county hospitals "dump" their moribund and "socially problematic" patients. Half of them are in a social crisis because they have no relatives who could take care of them at home. In such cases, the family physician sees no other alternative than to "medicalize" the patient's social situation and send the patient to a hospital or university clinic. The disadvantage of being in a hospital is that the longer an elderly person stays there, the less is the chance for rehabilitation. Since there are no geriatric wards or geriatric consultations to assess the overall well-being of the old, they are sent from one department to another to arrive at some kind of diagnosis. Nor is there much incentive, even in what we often call our "market-oriented health care system," to treat the old.

Clearly, Hungary needs to increase the number of geriatric wards and train more geriatricians, but at this point, no Hungarian university does this. Obviously, we need a good home care system and nursing homes as well, which could relieve the burden of the social homes—whose purpose is not nursing old people—and could provide what such homes should primarily provide: nursing care for those, for example, who lack mobility or are confined to a bed.

Economy and Morality

There is a strong tendency in our society to blame every social ill on the lack of money, especially in the field of health care. Yet tremendous waste of financial and personnel resources goes hand in hand with a lack of elementary conditions that could significantly increase the quality of life of those who are under the care of our social institutions. The lack of social support and skilled long-term care facilities, for example, means that beds in acute-care hospitals are being used to solve what are fundamentally social, rather than medical, problems. And while special luxury apartments are built for prominent leaders of the previous Communist era, public care facilities are in disarray. The buildings, for example, are unsuitable—overcrowded, with an inadequate number of rest rooms, bells to ask for help, or facilities for rehabilitation. The lack of devices that would make bathing and eating much easier also presents problems. But it is also a waste when certain diagnostic exams are repeated endlessly and when medical universities buy expensive Cadillacs, paintings, and extravagant furniture to impress visitors.

The differentiated salary system could also be considered irrational and immoral, since those who keep the health care system going—primary-care physicians, midlevel clinicians and hospital doctors, nurses, highly skilled assistants, dieticians, and cooks—are extremely underpaid, while those on the top of the hierarchy are in many cases significantly overpaid. The former receive about $150 to $200 per month, while the latter enjoy a salary around $1500 to $2000 per month. In many cases, salaries are adjusted to status and position, not to the actual work one performs.

The institutions are very much understaffed in specialists and skilled nurses. While there are about forty thousand people in public care institutions, the number of skilled nurses is only a little over four thousand. In the county of Baranya in southern Hungary on the Croatian border, for example, there are only eighteen nurses for every one hundred patients. This dramatic shortage of nurses is due to extremely low salary and the classic stereotype of nurses as handmaidens or even slaves to physicians. Thus, it is not rare that hospitals and/or wards have to be closed down because of a shortage of nurses. In fact, cardiac surgery in Budapest recently had to be discontinued because of a lack of skilled assistants and nurses. The country does train enough nurses, but they usually find employment outside the health care system or social institutions. In many social homes there are also no full-time physicians, dieticians, or physio- and psychotherapists. Yet Hungary is one of the leading nations in the world in the ratio of physicians to population.

In the population generally, the pauperization of retired people is rapidly increasing, as in all post-Communist countries. Under the one-party state system, salaries were established on an extremely low level, but the paternalistic socialist state added many social benefits to them: cheap rent; state-subsidized transportation, sport and cultural services, utilities, food prices, and even haircuts; low-interest loans; free health care; and drugs. All these have gone. Within our institutional care of the elderly, however, there is a system of providing one free meal a day, subsidized by the local government for those retired people whose pension is very low and who are not in social homes. Many aged people live on the cheapest food available. One wonders if such poverty can ever be accepted and tolerated with dignity.

State Paternalism and Individual Autonomy

The state paternalism of the former regime has deeply penetrated the whole texture of Hungarian society. Medical paternalism, which happily coexisted with state paternalism, has a much longer history, and therefore it is hard to tell which has had a stronger impact on the everyday lives of citizens. There is not much in life that old people can control, though it is well known that "a sense of control over one's life is associated with numerous positive outcomes, including improved health status."[4] Those who are better off financially, however, do enjoy a certain control. According to surveys, the higher one's pension, the more one's individual rights are respected.

That most, if not all, old people would consider it important not to be treated as persons in their second childhood doesn't necessarily mean that from time to time paternalistic behavior on the part of the care provider is not desired or accepted, of course. The line between justifiable and unjustifiable paternalism should be drawn when competent people reject contempt for their autonomy. The traditional model of extreme paternalism, in which an adult person is degraded to the status of an obedient child or to a passive puppet, is a serious violation of human dignity and autonomy.

Stories about social homes are frequent in Hungarian newspapers and journals, with headlines like "The Home of Beaten Old People" or "Drug Experiments on the Elderly." These stories demonstrate not simply unjustified paternalism but also the all-too-common kinds of maltreatment elderly people receive in many places around the world. A scandal that included the handcuffing of a former member of parliament illustrates well the conditions in some of the social homes in the country. The story revealed a range of abuses at the home involved, with allegations of experimentation on elderly residents and charges that residents were terrorized and subjected to physical violence. The elderly residents had been complaining for a long time, writing letters to various places, but it was learned that their letters were never delivered.[5] Investigations were hampered by the fact that residents were too sedated to be interviewed. Several residents committed or attempted to commit suicide. Such cases illustrate the general lack of professional and social control that makes it possible for caregivers and others in authority to abuse their power, a problem not by any means unique to institutional care.

As mentioned earlier, the opportunities for rehabilitation in social homes are very limited. Not only are the physical facilities generally not available— even the planning of buildings is inadequate for any meaningful rehabilitation— but there are too few specialists and skilled nurses. The lack of rehabilitation services may account in part for the widespread use of extensive medication, especially sedatives, although the "official" explanation is that the elderly suffer from many diseases. According to some estimates, drug consumption by the elderly accounts for about 25 percent of all medical costs in Hungary, a figure that corresponds with many other nations' drug use. A survey of drug use in the social homes of the county of Baranya showed that about 37 percent of residents take four to six kinds of drugs daily and 18.1 percent of residents take seven or more kinds. In the town of Pécs the average is ten to thirteen kinds of drugs. The elderly themselves often have a blind trust in medication, and relatives frequently demand that drugs be given to elderly residents.[6]

Social Homes and the Quality of Life

Family ties are the most important factor for the well-being of the elderly. Filial love cannot be legislated, of course, and moral obligations in families run deeper than the law. The law should, however, protect the elderly from financial exploitation and brutality by immoral family members. In Hungary there are laws compelling negligent children to provide care for their needy parents. Naturally, the coercive nature of the law makes even abused or neglected parents highly reluctant to ask the justice system for help, and thus these laws are rarely applied. All too often our social homes are crowded by visitors at the time residents receive their pension; the children or grandchildren take away the remaining money from their parents or grandparents. Nevertheless, these old people talk about their "wonderful" families till the next visit. For them nothing substitutes for the visits of relatives.

Even parents who showed great care and concern for their children throughout their lives may face a lonely and degrading old age. There are many stories of well-to-do sons and daughters who, rather than provide modest financial assistance, will do no more than collect free or subsidized meals and deliver them to their parents or who seek to place aging parents in psychiatric wards to avoid the burdens of caring for them, even when those burdens are not strenuous. For some, it seems that a little understanding and a few kind words are too much to ask.

Pets can help compensate for the lack of a family or the lack of a loving family. More and more elderly people keep some kind of animal that gives them company and someone to talk to and to take care of. It relieves some of the anxiety caused by loneliness, and it might be interpreted as a kind of solidarity with someone who has also been abandoned. But social homes forbid keeping pets, and it would only be possible in very few places.

The monotonous and overly regimented daily life in the social homes slowly makes the person indifferent to all that is going on around her. And as hearing, sight, and other capacities diminish, many tend to withdraw into themselves. Those who are very rarely or not at all visited may feel entirely abandoned and find no meaning in their lives.[7] The lack of love and the ever-increasing existential difficulties almost force many old people to turn to self-destruction. In Hungary the suicide rate among the elderly is very high even in comparison with the national rate, which already is one of the highest in the world. The annual rate of suicide attempts among the elderly is around three hundred per one hundred thousand and seems to be highest among the semiliterate who see no way of spending their lives usefully. When self-esteem and personal identity are gone, then comes the desire to die.

There is in Hungary a legally allowed form of care called "contract care." It means that in exchange for physical care or regular financial support, an individual—usually young or middle-aged—will inherit the assets and belongings of an old couple or single person after they die. Some gerontologists call these "contracts for death," considering them the most unethical device in the society. There are no statistics to show that abuses have occurred under such contracts, but they do risk leaving the old at the mercy of greedy fortune hunters.

A Promising Future?

What prospects does the future hold for the elderly in Hungary? Nowadays, after our radical political changes, we are "building" capitalism: an open-market system with private enterprise, unemployment, inflation, and high taxation. The old suffer most, since their pensions do not keep up with rising prices. There are, however, some positive signs too. A number of organizations, churches, and private foundations now provide home care for the elderly. Local governments also make some efforts to finance both home and institutional care, though their resources are limited because of many other serious problems they have to solve. And those who are financially more stable can turn to the private social homes that have also appeared on the scene. There are already more than twenty such enterprises in Hungary. They seem—or at least claim— to provide humane and homelike care suited to the individual's needs; full-time physicians and even beauticians and herbalists are on staff. The national government, recognizing the plight of the elderly, is trying to do something for them as well but is unable or unwilling to relieve the main burdens that they face in their daily lives. The government makes gestures toward the old, such as free public transportation or, in some ways more helpful perhaps, waiving the monthly television fee for people over the age of seventy.

For the state-run social institutions, there is less and less outside help. Earlier, in the Communist era, the so-called social brigades had given consider-able help to them. Not only financial help but humanistic as well. Members of such brigades did repair work, beautified parks and grounds, donated TVs and radios, visited the residents, and organized programs for them. The Young Pioneers (a Communist children's organization) had also supported the elderly by putting on entertainment programs and organizing birthday parties. This kind of altruism or ideological window dressing, whatever one calls it, was encouraged and rewarded as a proper display of good Communist behavior. All these have gone, and so far there is hardly any replacement.

Social scientists could help ease the situation for the elderly both by documenting their plight for the public and by finding solutions to many of the problems they face. Ethicists and philosophers are able to point out, for example, those human dimensions of the institutional care of the elderly that could be very much improved without significant financial investment. They could influence public opinion and policy makers in many respects, including attitudes toward the old (ranging from indifference to overtreatment) and priorities for resource allocation. They could bring the attention of the young to the need to prepare themselves for their old age. They could also contribute to the elderly's quality of life by providing both visions for the future and interpretations of the unavoidable changes taking place in our society today, in a way that translates the ivory-tower language into the colloquial terms of everyday morality. In fact, I would argue that philosophers and ethicists have a much greater responsibility than others to contribute moral insights for daily living. Ideas about the achievement of a happy old age—life fulfillment versus disillusionment—intergenerational coexistence, the limits and growth of one's potential, loneliness, and suicide should all be the terrain of the philosopher and ethicist.

To give a personal example, when my book on euthanasia was published ten years ago, a reader wrote appealing to me to assist her commit suicide or at least give her advice how she might do it herself or enlist a physician to help her. I had great difficulty composing an answer, but among other things, I asked her why she would want to deprive her children of the opportunity to care for her when she became old and seriously ill. Why should she come only to the conclusion that she would be a great burden on her family? Why not give her children the chance to put their gratitude to the test? As it turned out, her children displayed a wonderful sense of filial obligation and pulled her through her most difficult period. She is still alive, and we have kept a regular correspondence ever since. Of course, that may seem only a rather trivial example of how an ethicist could help point to various alternatives that may influence and enhance the quality of life of many people. Nevertheless, I am convinced that the public good can be significantly served by philosophers and ethicists disseminating ideas that can be of practical use at all levels of society.

Despite the very real difficulties in providing care for the elderly, neither scientists, nor philosophers, nor professional caregivers can allow themselves to be pessimistic. The responsibility is just too great to permit apathy, not because we might all reach an old age and should be assured better circumstances but because it is our inherent obligation to be the voice of all those who are at the boundary of our human community.[8]

REFERENCES

1. Hans-Georg Gadamer, "Ujraeled a Gyermekkor" (The revival of childhood), *Nepszabadsag,* 10 April 1993 p. 32; translated from *Die Zeit,* 26 March 1993, by Zsuzsa Glavina.

2. Laszlo Vertes, "Mindennapi Gerontologia" (Everyday gerontology), *Nepszabadsag,* 16 May 1990, p. 9.

3. Agota Horvath, *A Szocialis Otthon* (The social home) (Budapest: MTA Sociological Research Institute, 1988), p. 226.

4. Nancy S. Jecker and Donnie J. Self, "Medical Ethics in the 21st Century: Respect for Autonomy in Care of the Elderly Patient," *Journal of Critical Care* 6, no. 1 (1991): 47.

5. "Megvert Oregek Othhona" (The home of the beaten old people), editorial, *168 Oram,* 27 August 1991, pp. 22–23.

6. Maria Kopp and Arpad Skrabski, "The Hungarian Psychic State" (in Hungarian) (Budapest: Vegeken Foundation, 1992), p. 122.

7. Judit Novothy and Zoltanne Torma, "Szocialis Gondoskodas Baranya Megyeben" (Social care in the county of Baranya: Conclusions of a survey), unpublished Hungarian government document, 1988, pp. 19–21.

8. The author gratefully acknowledges the support of the Hungarian Scientific Research Fund. Research for this paper was conducted under grant number OTKA 28.

W. ANDREW ACHENBAUM

From Generation to Generation: Why U.S. Health Care Reform Is So Difficult in the Twentieth Century

The health care system should respond to the unique needs of each stage of life, sharing benefits and burdens fairly across the generations.

—*President Clinton's health security plan, 1993*

Every day there is a new push to get people to believe there is a crisis.

—*Sen. Robert Dole (R-Kansas)*

We don't have a health care crisis in this country.

—*Sen. Daniel Patrick Moynihan (D-New York)*

Health care reform now heads the U.S. domestic agenda. This generation of policy makers may be less successful than its predecessors, however, in effecting major changes. Current players now have different priorities in mind. Some see government as the only institution capable of providing universal coverage for all Americans—a goal that has eluded U.S. reformers for nearly a century. Others have made the containment of rampant inflation in the health care industry their primary objective. Since they embrace divergent policy assumptions, protagonists rarely use the same calculus in figuring costs, fiscal and otherwise.

And yet, despite all of the words uttered in support of various competing proposals and lawmakers' genuine efforts to talk about the basics, no major politician has fully articulated how profoundly population aging is going to alter present health care arrangements. No one has bluntly acknowledged that change is inevitable even if no legislation were enacted. The existing system was designed to deal with the nation's acute health care needs. Americans go to hospitals when they are *really* sick: they hope to save their lives by checking in, but they also know that they might never check out. Older patients by and large are treated like everybody else, though special programs were created entitling the aged to certain services and benefits that did not upset prevailing arrangements for the rest of the population.

By the middle of the next century, however, specialists will have much larger populations of patients over seventy-five. Geriatrics will no longer be a marginal specialty. Addressing the chronic ailments and functional incapacities of aging men and women will be the major concern of U.S. medicine. A new agenda will necessitate different institutional arrangements. Without reform, structural and cultural lags are inevitable. Yet in current debates politicians eschew such talk about future scenarios.

President Clinton's reform model was based on managed competition. Public or quasi-public health care alliances will negotiate various options for large groups of consumers. To provide information about each plan's cost and quality of care, an innovative nationwide gathering and evaluating of data outcomes would be established.[1] The president's plan was very complicated, and he expressed readiness to negotiate about everything except universal coverage. As Clinton appealed to various interest groups, he asked their support in demanding a wider array of services. Thus, in a speech before the National Council on the Aging, Clinton urged senior citizens and their advocates to demand that the often staggering price of prescription drugs be covered. Mindful of costs, the president did not say that he himself would include that provision in his final package.[2]

Key members of both parties, such as Senators Dole and Moynihan, resist anything so grandiose. They fear that implementing major health care reforms will cause the federal deficit to go further out of control. The concern is legitimate. Recently health care has been absorbing an additional 1 percent of the net domestic product every two and a half years. U.S. citizens spend more per capita than people in other advanced industrial countries. Despite smaller outlays, Canadians seem more satisfied with the quality of their care and their financial arrangements than their neighbors to the south.[3] Proposals to rationalize the system, claim conservatives, will increase an already bloated federal bureaucracy to nightmarish proportions. "Yes, there are problems," declared the Republican congressional leadership. Few discount the plight of 38.5 million Americans without health insurance in 1992 or the fact that the number of people covered under *employment-based* plans (such as Clinton proposes) declined even as pressure for health care reform mounted. "But there's not an emergency that requires a complete overhaul of the medical system."[4] The current debate is not drawn along Manichean lines. Rather, it pits visions of justice and fairness against fears that reforms may prove more costly and cumbersome than maintaining the status quo.

Promoting "the general welfare" is tough in a country where progress is measured incrementally. Advances occur in fits and turns; watersheds alternate with retrenchments. "The two parties which divide the state, the party of Conservatism and that of Innovation are very old. . . . Reform is affirmative, conservatism negative," Ralph Waldo Emerson observed in 1841. One set of reformers, responding to a (real or imagined) crisis, seeks to transform the status quo for the common good. In due course another set of political leaders, in reaction, tries to consolidate gains by curbing perceived excesses. In this dialectic, "innovation is the salient energy," opined the nation's leading nineteenth-century philosopher. "Conservatism the pause on the last movement."[5]

Reformism's ebb and flow was not a uniquely American characteristic; liberals fought conservatives everywhere. But the imagery that Emerson used to differentiate the two camps is revealing: "The conservative assumes sickness is a necessity, and his social frame is a hospital. . . . Reform converses with possibilities, perchance with impossibilities."[6] Furthermore, Emerson claimed that U.S. politics had generational underpinnings. Fresh ideas came from new blood, from reformers surmounting old ways and vested interests—"rest, conservatism, appropriation, inertia; not newness, not the way onward."[7] Partisan battles here are ideological, waged by forward-looking members of a rising generation against the elderly guardians of the established order. "I bring it home to the private heart, where all such questions must have their final arbitrament," Emerson declared. "How will every strong and generous mind choose its ground—with the defenders of the old? or with the seekers of the new? Which is the state which promises to edify a great, brave, and beneficent man; to throw him on his resources, and tax the strength of his character? On which part will each of us find himself in the hour of health and of aspiration."[8] Emerson looked for the reformer, but he knew well the power of conservatism over human nature.

Sometimes, of course, members of the same cohort represented the interests of innovation and conservatism. Debating among themselves a few decades earlier, for instance, members of the Revolutionary generation anticipated the contrapuntal logic that Emerson described. The Founding Fathers wrestled with how to balance the creative policy recommendations advanced by leaders coming into their own and the prudent voices of those who valued the steady hand of tradition. From the late 1780s until his death, Thomas Jefferson stressed that each generation had "the right to direct what is the concern of themselves alone, and to declare the law of that direction . . . to make the Constitution what they think will be best for themselves." Jefferson wrote in a letter in 1816 that the Constitution should make provisions for its own revision every nineteen or twenty years, "so that it may be handed on, with periodical repairs, from generation to generation, to end of the time."[9]

James Madison, in contrast, stressed the importance of continuity in transferring rights and responsibilities from generation to generation. "There seems then to be a foundation in the nature of things, in the relation which one generation bears to another, for the *descent* of obligation from one to another," Madison wrote to his neighbor at Monticello in 1790. "Equity requires it . . . [and] mutual good is promoted by it."[10] Revolutionary times surely occasioned new forms of comity. Yet the author of *Federalist Paper* 10 also acknowledged humans' innate capacity for selfishness and opportunism. Thus Madison relied on "traditional" conventions—instilling a sense of duty in the citizenry, honoring contracts that were legitimately made by representative governments—to dilute the naivete of political neophytes and to mitigate the Establishment's abuse of power.

At still other critical moments in our history, U.S. politicians have muted inter- and intragenerational disagreements over policy differences. Lawmakers in the depths of the Great Depression emphasized that "relief, reform, and reconstruction" actually offered the best way to preserve the core of the American experiment. Thus, in bringing together experts to draft social-security legislation, Franklin Delano Roosevelt declared: "Our task of reconstruction does not require the creation of new and strange values. It is rather the finding of the way once more to known, but to some degree forgotten, ideals and values. If the means and details are in some instances new, the objectives are as permanent as human nature."[11] The landmark Social Security Act of 1935 passed because it broadly satisfied what Arthur M. Schlesinger, Jr., called the nation's "vital center."

Social Security's transgenerational thrust appealed to many constituencies. Provisions for the indigent, the blind, and the elderly, as well as the funds earmarked for research and training, were all designed to give citizens new entitlements. The measure buttressed the traditional support that children owed their parents while enabling future generations to save for their retirement years. "It is my hope that soon the United States will have a national system under which no needy man or woman within our borders will lack a minimum old-age pension that will provide adequate food, adequate clothing and adequate lodging to the end of the road and without having to go to poorhouse to get it," FDR declared to members attending a Teamsters convention in 1940. "I look forward to a system . . . [that] will enable those who have faithfully toiled in any occupation to build up additional security for their old age which will allow them to lie in comfort and happiness."[12] Yet the president's chief advisors stressed that there were limits to program expansion, which required policy makers to be prudent. "The pattern cannot be larger than the cloth," observed J. Douglas Brown, who was one of the chief architects of the old-age provisions in the 1935 legislation. "The protection of the aged must not be at the expense of adequate protection of dependent children, the sick, the disabled, or the unemployed."[13]

FDR's blue-ribbon panel realized that illness was one of the major causes of economic insecurity. By their estimates, one-third to one-half of all dependency in the United States in "normal times" stemmed from the economic consequences of illness. Massive unemployment and cutbacks in services during the Depression, moreover, reduced the access of lower-income workers and their families to physicians and health care institutions. Yet the legacy of an earlier generation of reformers was hardly encouraging. On the one hand, the Progressives had succeeded in securing legislation to compensate against income losses due to industrial accidents. On the other hand, politicians in the 1910s had failed to enact compulsory insurance against sickness. In the process, they had lost the support of the medical establishment, who branded governmental intervention as a form of socialism. Hence New Deal reformers were content to set the stage for innovation:

> Insurance against the costs of sickness is neither new nor novel. In the United States we have had a long experience with sickness insurance both on a nonprofit and commercial basis. Both forms have been inadequate with respect to the protection they furnish, and the latter—commercial insurance—has in addition been too expensive for people of small means. Voluntary insurance holds no promise of being much more effective in the near future than it has been in the past.[14]

After deciding not to include health care insurance in its omnibus legislation, the Committee on Economic Security, as a "first and most inexpensive step in furnishing economic security against illness," requested funds to prevent sickness. Grants-in-aid were to provide public-health services in areas where none existed. (In 1933, only a sixth of the nation's counties had full-time health supervision.) Funds were allocated to train more personnel. (Only 21 percent of the existing local departments were providing "a satisfactory minimum" standard in dealing with health-related problems.)

Noting that "nearly every large and industrial country of the world except the United States has applied the principle of insurance to the economic risks of illness,"[15] the committee charted a pragmatic agenda for their successors.

They envisioned a health system that pooled risks. Policy makers set a 4.5 percent cap on a family's contribution for medical coverage. In return, eligible beneficiaries could expect to receive cash for lost wages and/or in-kind medical and health services. The medical profession would control personnel and services and negotiate fees. Services would be administered on a statewide basis, with the federal government establishing national standards and providing necessary subsidies.

Philosophically and structurally, the committee's blueprint for health care reform meshed with the logic and form of its Social Security Act. Private interests buttressed public aims: Blue Cross plans, community-based health care centers, and life insurance companies were to supplement and eventually replace friendly societies and "sickness funds" as vehicles for improving the access of middle-class patients to hospitals, and vice versa. Capitalizing on federalism's appeal, the architects provided checks and balances in establishing lines of authority for national, state, and local jurisdictions. Channeling health insurance options through employment, moreover, promised to protect providers against excessive public regulation and to rely on the competitive forces of the marketplace to contain costs and reduce abuses. Finally, the proposed health insurance scheme gave citizens a right to coverage against risks associated with sickness while holding them responsible for bearing some of the burdens. (The parallels with Clinton's reform package should be manifest.)

As was the case with New Deal income maintenance programs, age-specific differences in people's health status were acknowledged but not accentuated. Modern technology and medical interventions, the experts noted, had conquered many childhood illnesses and increased life expectancy at birth. Still, gains were uneven. "The mortality of adults of middle and older ages has not been appreciably diminished," the committee reported. "With the changing age composition of our population the task of health conservation must be broadened to include adults as well as children."[16] Reformers ultimately hoped to reduce every cohort's risk by providing universal coverage over the life course. Faced with limited resources and considerable opposition, they opted for an incremental approach, addressing needs that could be remedied with the least political cost.

New federal investments, incentives, and rulings restructured the nation's health care institutions after World War II. The Veterans Administration, which operated the largest hospital system in the United States, became the major training site for physicians and nurses. The National Institutes of Health grew into the world's largest center for biomedical research. The Hill-Burton Act (1946) provided billions for hospital construction, which increased the number of beds available in low-income states and Middle America. Changes in the tax code during the 1950s exempted employers' contributions to health benefit plans. By 1954, 12 million union members and their 17 million dependents enjoyed Blue Cross/Blue Shield coverage. Some workers took advantage of prepaid group-practice options like the Kaiser plan.[17]

As conservatives and innovators in each Congress haggled over details, additional health care benefits were gradually extended to certain classes of Social Security recipients. The 1950 amendments provided means-tested payments to the disabled. Broader disability provisions were added during the Eisenhower years for those too young to retire but incapable of staying in the labor force. The Kerr-Mills Act (1960) allocated funds for people not on public relief who could not pay for necessary medical treatments. Each legislative victory heightened public interest in medical insurance, which in turn presaged another wave of health care innovation in Washington.

"We can—we must—strive now to ensure the availability and accessibility to the best health care for all Americans regardless of age or geography or economic status," proclaimed Lyndon Baines Johnson, setting a major goal for his Great Society.[18] A new generation of reformers focused on the needs of the elderly, who constituted the poorest and sickest segment of society. In 1965 the president signed Medicare into law. The measure extended hospital insurance to Social Security beneficiaries and featured a voluntary plan (originally costing participants only $36 per year) to cover physicians' bills. Seizing on the historical significance of Public Law 98-97, LBJ flew to Independence, Missouri, so that he could sign the measure in the presence of Harry S. Truman, who a political generation earlier had valiantly fought for a government health insurance plan. Just as old-age assistance in 1935 had been considered a necessary complement to old-age insurance, so too Medicaid (which provided medical services for welfare recipients of all ages) was enacted in the shadow of Medicare.

The very effectiveness of engaging in the politics of incrementalism accentuated the importance of the popular Social Security apparatus for initiating subsequent reform initiatives. Social Security amendments in 1972 permitted reimbursements for kidney dialysis and transplants, chiropractic and podiatry services under Medicare, and liberalized Medicaid payments for nursing home care. These 1972 amendments, however, also signaled Congress's first efforts to limit health care outlays. Medicare authorized certain services on a capitation basis and established review boards to monitor quality and utilization of resources. Medicaid permitted states to impose copayment requirements on recipients.[19]

As stagflation and political crises deepened people's mistrust of government, reformers yielded to the forces of conservatism. Ford and Carter's calls for greater stringency floundered. Ronald Reagan was the first president to succeed in framing the health care debate in economic terms. Congress, however, was loath to consider measures that might hurt the poor and the elderly. The Catastrophic Coverage Act (1988) provided new benefits in a seemingly budget-neutral fashion. But Congress repealed the measure two years later when faced with considerable backlash from the very constituency it meant to help. That relatively affluent senior citizens were unwilling to pay for catastrophic coverage exposed *intra*generational cleavages in the electorate.

The fight over catastrophic insurance was symptomatic of larger fiscal woes, structural dysfunction, and stereotypic reasoning. Increases in life expectancy were a source of national pride. Population aging nonetheless was scary—it raised the spectre of additional burdens. Sophisticated medical technology saved lives, yet it also prolonged the process of dying. On purely budgetary grounds, facts did not always square with intuitive sense: "People who die of ill behavior at, say, age sixty are probably less of a financial 'burden' on the health care system than those supposedly more virtuous persons who live, and so continue to incur costs, well into their eighties," noted Brookings analyst Joseph White.[20] Treating Alzheimer's patients costs more on average than illnesses that lead to death associated with smoking. Comparing U.S. life expectancies with those of people in other countries did indicate that buying higher-quality medical care for life-threatening illnesses has gained Americans years. Yet few people really believe that performing quadruple coronary bypasses on octogenarians in an effort to prolong their lives a few weeks (at best) should be automatically covered by federal programs already under strain.

So while voters and politicians want the very best for Mom, most acknowledge that rationing already occurs in the U.S. health care system and that more will have to occur in the future unless Americans are prepared to pay more. (In 1960, Americans paid roughly 70 percent of their health care expenditures out of their own pockets; by 1991, the percentage had declined to about 40 percent. Meanwhile, private insurance payments doubled.)[21] Inflation in the health care industry far outstripped Congress's ability to contain Medicare and Medicaid costs. It once was considered good politics to link medical insurance to Social Security eligibility. For more than a decade, the economics of health care no longer has seemed analogous to Federal Insurance Contribution Act (FICA) accounting. And while most U.S. citizens are basically satisfied with their personal health care arrangements, the percentage of those who think the system needs reform rose from 19 percent to 42 percent between 1987 and 1991.[22]

Significantly, however, the greatest impediment to U.S. health care reform in the 1990s is neither fiscal, nor political, nor social. The challenge is institutional. For all its virtues and deficiencies, the thorniest problems besetting the current system is that in orientation and delivery, it too sharply delineates acute and chronic disease. Institutions have adapted historically to age-specific changes in death rates from heart diseases, malignant neoplasms, and cerebrovascular diseases.[23] Primary care, immunization, and low-tech rehabilitation programs, in contrast, are rarely considered significant features of our overall health care network—despite their vital importance in elder care. Nor is old age what it used to be. People turning sixty-five do not suddenly embark on that slippery slope from good to bad health. They are more likely to experience a variety of transitions: setbacks due to broken hips, followed by improved functioning; chronic ailments worsened by heart attacks, with recovery facilitated by social-service interventions that make independence possible.

Current events, moreover, require us to rethink whether the acute orientation that dictates how health care is delivered in the United States optimally addresses the needs of people *under* sixty-five. The AIDS crisis, for example, belies any facile association of death with senescence. Everybody has seen photographs of gaunt faces of victims in their prime who now look "old." In addition to suffering from multiple chronic impairments, their bodies' functions and capacities are cruelly diminished with each bout of pneumonia or cancer.

In a different realm, the passage of the Americans with Disabilities Act (1992), which prevents discrimination from any program underwritten by federal dollars, is already affecting the entire health care enterprise. Yet here too, structural lags persist. Disability insurance is the least important component of Old Age, Survivors, Disability, and Hospital Insurance (OASDHI), yet Social Security is the most important part of our nation's disability policy. Disability is the primary reason workers retire early, yet its definition eludes lawyers, bureaucrats, scholars, and employers.[24] Disability is a fuzzy concept because morbidity patterns vary greatly by age, race, and gender. "If we are really concerned about improving health status and public health," observes John Rother, chief policy spokesperson for the American Association of Retired Persons, "then we need to think about integrated systems that look at chronic care, that take into account the role of prevention in public health as much as, or even more than, the need to integrate the acute care parts of the delivery system."[25]

Reconfiguring the conceptual connections among aging, disability, and long-term care necessitates a reordering of the status quo. We can no longer build on acute-care models. The history of pediatrics offers practical lessons for developing cross-disciplinary geriatric paradigms but hardly resolves the issues of patients' autonomy and choices. On what grounds should one decide to ration high-tech medical resources solely on the basis of age? If not chronology, then what criterion—likely life expectancy? functionality? wealth?—is more appropriate?

As Americans acknowledge the limits of their capacities, they will need to make explicit their decision making about resource allocations. Alas, President Clinton's health security plan did not really go far enough. Senators Dole and Moynihan can temporize, but incremental tinkering no longer suffices. *This* generation must squarely face the challenges and opportunities presented by societal aging. The times demand that advocates of innovation respect "traditional" values—freedom of choice, respect for privacy—as we imagine our future selves. Alas, if past is prologue, then conservatism's sway may blind us to our responsibility to face that future. If so we may squander our last chance to effect meaningful reform in the U.S. health care system for some time to come.

REFERENCES

1. Note the parallel between this proposal and the need for governmental information-gathering services set forth in "What Do We Owe the Elderly?" special supplement, *Hastings Center Report* 24, no. 2 (1994): S1–S12, at S5.

2. For a concise view of the Clinton package around spring 1994, see William S. Custer, "Reforming the Health Care Delivery System," *Employee Benefit Research Institute Special Report* 21 (April 1994): 8–22. The president's speech, delivered in Washington on 27 April 1994, is available from the White House.

3. Statistics from Henry J. Aaron, "Paying for Health Care," *Domestic Affairs* no. 2 (Winter 1993–94): 23–26.

4. "What Health Crisis?" *National Journal*, 29 January 1994. The quotations from Dole and Moynihan in the epigraph also come from this article.

5. Ralph Waldo Emerson, "The Conservative," in *Nature: Addresses and Lectures* (Boston: Houghton Mifflin, 1903), pp. 293, 298, 303, 297.

6. Ibid., p. 313.

7. Quoted in David Hackett Fischer, *Growing Old in America* (New York: Oxford University Press, 1977), p. 113.

8. Ibid., p. 322.

9. Letter of Thomas Jefferson to Samuel Kerchival, 12 July 1816, in *The Life and Writings of Thomas Jefferson,* ed. William Peden (New York: Modern Library, 1944), pp. 675–76.

10. Quoted in Drew McCoy, *The Last of the Fathers* (New York: Cambridge University Press, 1989), p. 58.

11. Franklin Delano Roosevelt, "Message to Congress reviewing the broad objectives and accomplishments of the Administration," 8 June 1934, in Alan Pifer and Forrest Chisman, eds., *Report of the Committee on Economic Security of 1935,* 50th anniversary edition (Washington: National Conference on Social Welfare, 1985), p. 136.

12. *Franklin Delano Roosevelt Public Papers* (New York: Macmillan), 9: 411.

13. Quoted in W. Andrew Achenbaum, *Social Security: Visions and Revisions* (New York: Cambridge University Press, 1986), p. 35.

14. *Report of the Committee on Economic Security,* in Pifer and Chisman, *Report of the Committee,* p. 61.

15. Ibid. Provisions on pp. 62–63.

16. Ibid., p. 59.

17. Paul Starr, *The Social Transformation of American Medicine* (New York: Basic Books, 1983).

18. "Message to Congress on January 7, 1965," in *Public Papers of the Presidents of the United States: Lyndon B. Johnson, 1965* (Washington: Government Printing Office, 1966), 1: 13.

19. Achenbaum, *Social Security,* pp. 169–71.

20. Joseph White, "Redefining the Health Care Promise," *Domestic Affairs* no. 2 (Winter 1993–94): 233.

21. Helen C. Lazrenby, Katharine R. Levit, and Suzanne Lesch, "National Health Expenditures, 1991," *Health Care Financing Review* 14 (Winter 1992): 1–30.

22. Lawrence R. Jacobs and Robert Y. Shapiro, "The Duality of Public Opinion," *Domestic Affairs* no. 2 (Winter 1993–94): 251.

23. Frank L. Schick and Renee Schick, *Statistical Handbook on Aging Americans* (Phoenix: Oryx Press, 1994), chap. C; Institute of Medicine, *Health in an Older Society* (Washington: National Academy Press, 1985).

24. Eric R. Kingson and Edward D. Berkowitz, *Social Security and Medicare: A Policy Primer* (Westport, Conn.: Auburn House, 1993), pp. 137–40.

25. Quoted in the Employee Benefit Research Institute special report, *The Changing Health Care Delivery System* (Washington, D.C.: E.B.R.I., April 1994), p. 1.

A PROJECT REPORT BY
RUUD H. J. TER MEULEN, EVA TOPINKOVÁ, AND
DANIEL CALLAHAN

What Do We Owe the Elderly? Allocating Social and Health Care Resources

KEY RECOMMENDATIONS

1. *The highest future goal of medicine for the elderly should be a reduction in morbidity and disability and not an explicit effort to reduce mortality or increase average life expectancy. Old age is an inevitable human condition, one that should not be defined as a medical problem to be conquered or as a set of problems wholly amenable to medical or scientific solutions. Human beings will continue to age, to get sick, and to die.*

2. *The maintenance of a firm sense of moral solidarity between the generations has—in the face of competing and fragmenting pressures and uncertainty about the nature and extent of ethical obligation—become an urgent matter for social dialogue and refinement. The old will continue in great part to depend heavily upon the young, both for financial resources, conveyed by government through taxation or directly through the family, and for the personal care they receive from the young in the intimacy of family life.*

3. *An integrated set of priorities for young and old should be pursued as part of an effort to devise a fair and sensible allocation of resources between the generations and within the generations. The young and the old should work together to develop those priorities and be prepared to share equitably any limits on the use of resources that may be required.*

4. *The burden upon women in the care of the elderly that has marked informal caregiving in the past cannot and should not be sustained. This change will require a new strategy in the division of responsibility for informal care and the development of new government programs to nourish caregiving of this kind.*

5. *Active efforts should be undertaken to help the elderly to organize politically and to define and articulate their major needs collectively. A high priority in that effort* *should be to end the frequent separation of health and welfare programs and to make clear to the public and government that no sharp or meaningful lines can be drawn between the varied and overlapping needs of the elderly: social, economic, and medical.*

6. *A public dialogue on the significance of old age in the common life of society should be advanced through educational programs, the media, and joint governmental-private efforts. These efforts should encompass future possibilities for the elderly in the realms of work and leisure. Additional efforts should be fostered to help the elderly think through their personal meanings and goals.*

Barring accident or mischance, the majority of human beings in developed societies will move from youth through adulthood to old age. Even now there may be more surprises in store for those on the threshold of old age than for those already well advanced in years—a greater chance of living in good health into their nineties and, most remarkably for a growing number, beyond the age of 100. For those now in their middle years, the prospects are even more hopeful, consisting of healthier early years, increased preventive knowledge, and technological advances. In the twentieth century, life expectancy at birth has increased by over thirty years. And given the demographic surprises of recent decades, which have constantly exceeded all expectations of longevity, it is impossible even to speculate meaningfully on the prospects of the young and those just now being born.

Yet these great changes are beginning to bring with them some extremely troubling questions—social, economic, and medical:

- If a majority of elderly people, particularly those in their sixties and seventies, are healthy and vigorous, many are not; and by their eighties many more can expect to be burdened by some degree of chronic illness and disability.

- If there is more and more enthusiasm for extending the advantages of high-technology medicine to the elderly, the economic cost of that progress can be prodigious.

- If more of the elderly are able to continue working well past statutory retirement ages, economic obstacles in many societies that are beset with high unemployment rates for young people may not easily make that possible.

- If more elderly are able to maintain themselves in their homes with only a moderate degree of family assistance, there are fewer and fewer family members at home to provide that help.

- If more countries than ever are beginning to grasp the economic implications of an aging society and the need for increased and improved services, those same countries no less see growing taxpayer resistance to expensive welfare and health care programs.

The general dimensions of the problem of the elderly are well known. They include demographic projections, in every developed country, of a great increase in the number and proportion of the elderly over the next few decades, together with a corresponding and related decline in the number and proportion of younger people. The increase in the elderly is particularly notable for those over the age of eighty. Even in the short term, for the countries represented in this project, that group will increase by 15 to 30 percent between 1990 and the year 2000. Simply to maintain the level of services available in 1990, an increase of 10 to 15 percent in resources for home and institutional care will be needed—a daunting number in the face of pressures to hold down such spending in all countries. If the demographic and economic projections are run out through the years 2020 and 2030, when the present generation of middle-aged people has moved into the retirement age, the figures are all the more intimidating.

The governments of the developed countries have not been indifferent to these emerging demographic trends. None have wholly ignored them. Nonetheless, there is a remarkable degree of variation from one country to the next. Some display active government programs to improve the social, economic, and medical status of the elderly in the short run, but there are comparatively few efforts to begin preparing now for the almost certain pressures in the near future. Long-range planning, particularly bringing into that process the now young who will one day become the next generation of the old, is almost everywhere absent. Planning and even serious discussion about the future have not taken place although data and trends clearly foreshadow the kinds of problems and dilemmas almost certain to arise.

Even current programs and policies are erratic in dealing with those crises already present. Some countries that provide decent governmental programs reveal few and relatively weak efforts to organize voluntary programs for the elderly and to help them organize themselves as a political force. Some countries have strong acute-care medical programs for the elderly but much weaker social and long-term care programs. Some countries have begun serious efforts to find a more meaningful and dignified social place for the elderly, while in others the elderly seem mainly to be looked upon as a burden, the object of discrimination and stigmatization. It is not our intention to single out any particular country for praise or blame, and we recognize that some of the countries included in our study—particularly those in Central Europe—are only now coming out of the disastrous decades of Communist domination and have enormous problems to face in reforming their welfare and health care programs. (At the same time, to be sure, they have some enormous new opportunities.)

The Purpose of This Report

The purpose of this report is to present the reflections of an international research group that focused its attention on the moral problems of care for the elderly in the years ahead, in particular on the problem of an equitable and reasonable allocation of resources. By stressing the "moral" problems, we mean to call attention to an often neglected dimension of the public and professional discussion: the obligations owed to the elderly by individuals and society, the reciprocal obligations on the part of the elderly, and the ethical dilemmas that sensitive care for them cannot avoid. Most generally, we want to call attention to the often hidden value issues and considerations of a discussion that, in most countries, is restricted to economic and institutional arrangements only.

Our research group determined, at the outset, that the scope of its work would include both medical and more general welfare programs and that by "care for the elderly" we would encompass cultural, social, economic, and health perspectives. It is fair to say, however, that our report is comparatively more oriented toward the medical aspects of the problem. Five dimensions of the general issue were identified early in the project, and our investigations moved back and forth among them. They provide the basic ingredients of this report: (1) the meaning and significance of aging in contemporary society; (2) the goals of medicine and health care for the elderly; (3) balancing the needs of the young and the old—intergenerational obligations; (4) resource allocation and social priorities—setting limits; and (5) families, women, society, and long-term care. These five elements are developed at greater length and in greater detail in other publications that will result from this project.

At the heart of our common work and reflections were two interrelated goals. The first was to see if we could develop for the care of the elderly a moral and philosophical framework that could effectively serve to undergird public policy. How can society's obligations toward the elderly be best conceptualized and deployed to inform the day-to-day work of programs and policies for the elderly? The second goal was to see if some coherent integration of four important elements of a morally informed public policy could be achieved. They are: (1) to give a higher priority to the social and welfare needs of the elderly, together with a far greater emphasis on the reduction of morbidity than is now the case; (2) to better understand and make plausible to society the nature of the bonds that unite the young and the old and how those bonds can best be expressed ethically in devising programs for the elderly; (3) to grapple with the nature of family responsibility for the elderly at a time of great change in the nature of the family and in its possibilities for providing care; and (4) to see where the responsibility of the elderly for themselves fits into the picture at a time when new opportunities for the vitality and independence of the elderly are cast against a backdrop of tightened expenditures of government health and welfare programs designed to care for them.

To articulate those four elements in a slightly different way, our group was animated by a desire to see if we could discern a direction, even vision, for the future that would include an altered set of medical goals, a renewal of the bonds of solidarity between the generations, and a fresh negotiation of the tripartite relationship of obligations—of the elderly to care for themselves, of their families to care for them, and of government to see their care as a state obligation. We were also animated by a desire to see if the possibilities for some tragic dilemmas and conflicts in the future could be minimized, even averted if possible. They include (a) the potential for a conflict between the young and the old in their respective need for resources; (b) a morally agonizing gap between the possibilities of a medical improvement in the health of the elderly and a societal willingness or capacity to pay for them; and (c) terrible struggles within families over meeting the needs of elderly parents and spouses in the face of changing roles of women, the competing needs of children in the family, and a threatened reduction in government-provided resources to meet those pressures.

We cannot claim that we got to the bottom of this complex set of problems. They are difficult enough when taken individually, and all the more so when an effort is made to see them whole and together. Yet we hope that the six recommendations we make below, and the commentary accompanying them, suggest a fruitful direction for the future. We all need to know in what *general* direction we should be heading. To know at least that much, while it will not itself provide relief from the detailed complexities of good public policy, might bring to the task a coherent perspective and moral framework, and that would help.

A Necessary Prerequisite

Before moving on to our specific recommendations, it is necessary to underscore a prerequisite of good public policy for the elderly. As noted above, there is a significant variation from country to country in the attention paid to the elderly by government, and a considerable disparity in the type and quality of information gathered about them. There are two issues to be distinguished here. One of them is the necessity that a government signal, by its programs and priorities, the importance it attaches to the welfare of the elderly. Government activities on behalf of the elderly should be strong and highly visible, a sign of the seriousness of the commitment. This is critical for the elderly, who need continuing evidence that their worries and needs are accorded high-level attention. They must not feel neglected or forgotten, and even the symbolic effort on the part of government to give the agencies and departments charged with their welfare a place of prestige and prominence is an important step in that direction.

The other issue is how best to organize programs and policies for the elderly. Should they be centralized in one government program or be distributed among different departments and between the public and the private sectors? While a government centralization of programs can have some virtues and practical values, there is even more to be said for a variety of institutions and agencies, public and private. Centralization increases the likelihood of rigid and excessive bureaucracy. By contrast, a plurality of institutions offers the advantage of flexibility, different approaches and strategies for different issues, and greater responsiveness to particular problems. At the same time, however, there remains an important role for government in trying, formally and informally, to coordinate different programs and keep them in contact with each other and to provide oversight so that no important problems are overlooked. The coordination of federal and state programs, as well as such other institutions as universities, research institutes, and insurance companies, will be an important part of these efforts.

There is a major role that only government can suitably play, that of the collection and dissemination of data on the elderly and on those social and economic trends that affect their well-being. The collection of such information requires the legal powers and resources of government as well as the ability to look carefully at the overall picture of the welfare of the elderly. While there is a variation from country to country in the extent and sophistication of the data-collecting mechanisms and the data actually collected, some common gaps seemed evident. The most notable ones bear on the provision of health care outside institutions and on knowledge about informal care and services.

Even a determination of how much and what kind of medical and social-welfare resources the elderly consume is difficult if not impossible to reach in most countries. The relationship between costs in the health care sector and those in the social-service sector remains a mystery almost everywhere. So also does the relative proportion of funds spent on high-technology, acute-care medicine, on the one hand, and low-technology medical regimens and services, on the other. The fact that different countries, when they collect such information at all, do so in varied ways is perhaps understandable, given different traditions and forms of government. But it also bespeaks an absence, in the international community, of scientifically accepted and established methods of acquiring reliable and consistent information, a loss both to the countries themselves and to international communication and shared reform efforts. This problem is particularly urgent for the member states of the European Community, which are trying to unify their policies in various social areas. If governments lack good data, the possibilities of devising relevant and effective policies are seriously diminished. It is thus imperative that governments develop good systems for collecting and analyzing data on the elderly and that they make this information available to public and private agencies in a timely and useful manner.

Key Recommendations

We have six recommendations to make. They fall into two general classes: the first four bear on what we take to be the most urgent issues facing public policy in the future, and the final two on some necessary background conditions needed to deal with them.

> **Recommendation 1.** *The highest future goal of medicine for the elderly should be a reduction in morbidity and disability and not an explicit effort to reduce mortality or increase average life expectancy. Old age is an inevitable human condition, one that should not be defined as a medical problem to be conquered or as a set of problems wholly amenable to medical or scientific solutions. Human beings will continue to age, to get sick, and to die.*

Directly or indirectly, the perceived meaning and significance of old age will heavily determine resource allocation. They will also be complemented by medicine's understanding of its role and possibilities in care for the aged. Yet medicine has in modern times displayed a fundamental ambivalence about aging and the death that comes at its end. In one respect it understands well enough that aging is the fate of all organisms and that death is the inevitable endpoint of their life. Yet it seems no less true that scientific medicine—ambitious, hopeful, and expansionary in its goals—has come to separate aging and disease and illness and death. The aspiration of that medicine is to eliminate as many as possible of the diseases and harmful conditions hitherto correlated with aging and to cure those diseases that bring death.

This has been in many ways a highly successful venture. A large number of people can, with the aid of medicine, live long lives in relatively good health, remaining active and able to care for themselves. And the greater proportion of people who live long enough to achieve old age is still another sign of the success of that venture.

Yet that success, and especially the hope for still more, has come at a price. It has created an enormous bias in most health care systems toward those forms of medicine—especially hospital-based, acute-care medicine—aimed at curing disease and forestalling death. The power and prestige of contemporary medicine have come to reside in the search for medical cures and the use of high-technology, acute-care services to extend life. This potent trend, most pronounced since World War II, has inadvertently relegated to an inferior, second-best place the wide range of nursing, custodial, and rehabilitation services needed by the elderly when acute-care medicine can no longer help them. While some countries have paid lip service to a slogan that can be traced to the British National Health Service—"Adding life to years rather than years to life"—the gradual increase in the prestige of high-technology, lifesaving medicine and the rise in resources devoted to it have too often eclipsed that idea. It is still an important idea, one that needs to be kept as vigorously alive as possible and used to animate those programs that will indeed add "life to years."

Little prestige, inadequate resources, and much less research are directed toward improving or stabilizing the lives of those beyond the reach of high-technology medicine. A traditional part of the ethics of medicine, that of caring for those who cannot be cured, is sometimes forgotten altogether but more often starved of the resources necessary to make it efficacious and telling in the lives of the elderly.

This trend has been all the more unfortunate when taken in tandem with the increased burden of chronic disease and disability that have come to be the mark of modern old age. As mortality rates have declined, morbidity rates have increased. The effect of longer lives is, often enough, more sickness; those who would in the past have died can now be saved, but not necessarily made whole or well again.

A sensible and humane allocation of resources to the elderly in the future will have to work toward a much improved balance between curing and caring. It is curing that should, when economic pressure is strong, give way to caring, not the other way around. A medicine that can save lives but leave more sick and damaged people in its wake ironically can create even more problems than it solves, often sparing people a quick death but giving them, in its stead, a longer life marked by sickness and disability. Now is the time to recognize and act upon the sharply increased need to improve the quality of life of the elderly, and not simply to lengthen their lives.

Medicine cannot eliminate aging and death, only ameliorate their impact and shift their timing. Medicine should not be expected to conquer the decline of the human body, but only to soften its blows. The great frontier of health care for the elderly is a reduction, not in mortality rates, but in the morbidity and disability associated with aging. A public that has not been beguiled into thinking that medicine can conquer death, or all the causes of death, and that understands the inescapable fact of mortality needs to be fostered. An educated public will not so easily expect or demand what it cannot be given, nor be led to invest an unfair and excessive amount of social resources in struggling against the decline in bodily power and the increase in the threat of death that are part of growing old.

In stressing the necessity of achieving a better balance between cure and care, we do not mean to minimize the importance that new technological developments can have for the health of the elderly, whether for cure or care. Medical science will and should increase its knowledge of the underlying biology of aging, and some of that knowledge will lead to useful technological applications for the relief of illness and disease. At the same time, there is bound to be a continuation of a strong and important recent trend in the medical treatment of the elderly: the successful application to the elderly of diagnostic and therapeutic procedures originally developed with younger populations in mind. Advances in kidney dialysis and open-heart surgery provide two obvious illustrations of this trend. More recent developments of great importance are the technologies to facilitate home care. They will need evaluation no less than the technologies of hospitals and clinics. They have the potential both to relieve pressures on family members and also significantly to increase the costs of home care.

Yet it is imperative that there be a careful, scientifically solid evaluation of the use of medical technologies in the care of the old. In some countries that were part of our study there is a reasonable, well-founded concern that the elderly are not receiving the benefit of medical technologies that would be of value to them, whether for economic reasons or because of an outdated set of medical prejudices about what is appropriate treatment for the aged. In other countries, by contrast, the worry is just the opposite: that too much high-technology medicine is lavished upon the elderly without sufficient regard for the actual benefits to them. What seems obvious in both cases, however, is the urgent need for a careful assessment of medical technologies in the care and treatment of the elderly. The burgeoning international technology assessment movement, incorporating an effort to assess medical outcomes, needs be encouraged and financially supported. Which technologies, under what conditions, can be useful for maintaining the health and life of the elderly? Which technologies may be helpful but, because of their high costs, pose serious economic and moral dilemmas? There are too few answers to those questions at present. Hardly less important is the need to train those who care for the elderly in attending to the assessment information as it becomes available. Their own clinical judgment and local knowledge will need to be fleshed out, and sometimes altered, by more general scientific studies and information.

At the same time—and in the face of the developing technologies—the strong modern bias toward medicalizing the problem of aging needs forcefully to be fought. The prestige of medicine as a source of money, the medical legitimation of socially troubling conditions, and the success of medicine in dealing with a wide range of humanly vexing problems have made it tempting to see in medical thought and research a panacea to all social and individual problems. This can mean treating old age itself as a correctable disease, or using medical means, and medical prestige, as an umbrella under which to put all the problems of aging.

Good health care for the elderly requires many services and the help of many institutions that are not part of medicine at all. The economic and pension programs that can make such a direct difference in the living conditions of the elderly and a no less important indirect difference in the health of the elderly are outside medicine, and properly so. What is important is not to medicalize all the needs of the elderly, but to coordinate among a number of medical and nonmedical fields and services the full range of the needs of the elderly. To medicalize all such needs, or even a large proportion of them, communicates a wrong message about the meaning and place of aging in human life, tends to diminish the importance of nonmedical social services, and assigns to medicine the central role in improving the lives of the elderly—a role it should not have imposed upon it.

An increased emphasis on geriatric training for all health care workers that focuses on the social as well as medical needs of the elderly, together with an expansion and improvement of the field of geriatrics, would make an important contribution to improving the care of the aged.

Recommendation 2. *The maintenance of a firm sense of moral solidarity between the generations has—in the face of competing and fragmenting pressures and uncertainty about the nature and extent of ethical obligation—become an urgent matter for social dialogue and refinement. The old will continue in great part to depend heavily upon the young, both for financial resources, conveyed by government* *through taxation or directly through the family, and for the personal care they receive from the young in the intimacy of family life.*

An important characteristic of the developing countries of the world is the pyramid-shaped distribution of the different age groups, with a heavy predominance of the young and children at the bottom of the pyramid. The *developed* countries by contrast show an increasingly cylindrical pattern, with the number of the old coming to match the number of those under the age of eighteen. The implications of this pattern are alarming: a reduced number and proportion of young people will become heavily responsible for welfare and medical programs needed by the old.

This development poses two distinct challenges. One of them is practical: what kind of financing policies can be developed to ensure adequate resources for the elderly without placing insupportable burdens on the shoulders of the young? The other is moral: what is a fair and equitable way of politically apportioning the economic and social costs of providing adequate resources to the old? Behind that question lies still another: what are the moral obligations of the young to care for the old, both those in their own families and those who are strangers to them? Within families, it may be time and personal trouble that are more necessary than financial assistance; where the care of strangers is at stake, the obligation is likely to be discharged through the impersonal mechanism of taxation.

In the end, moreover, the practical and the moral cannot readily be separated. A workable practical system of allocating adequate resources to the elderly must command some significant degree of public support; otherwise the elderly will be neglected or given marginal resources only. The most likely motivating factor for decent public support will be the sense of moral obligation felt toward the old. But that sense will be greatly strengthened by a pervasive recognition that self-interested individual prudence has a vital role to play as well: we all get old and we are all at risk for the hazards of old age. It is not only someone else who is likely to need good policies and services; it is ourselves as well.

The traditional moral foundation for obligations to the elderly has been intergenerational reciprocity, the relatively simple notion that the old have duties toward the well-being of the young and the young, in turn, have duties toward the well-being of the old. The notion of gratitude, particularly within families, has been an important complementary or alternative foundation for obligation. The dependency of the young is matched by the dependency of the old. It is thus both fair and reasonable that the different age groups be prepared, when they are able, to provide resources for each other as required by the changing circumstances of their lives and the shifting of dependency status.

Yet the moral traditions of reciprocity are under many forms of subtle corrosion or outright attack. In some cases, the fragmentation and mobility of once intact families, closely bound to each other by virtue at least of proximity, has brought physical distance between young and old family members, thus making it harder to provide physical and emotional support. In other cases, the expectation in many welfare states that it is the role of government, not families, to provide the basic sustenance for the old has weakened the sense of personal obligation for the fate of an elderly family member. In a time of growing disillusionment with government, it is tempting for many groups in society to think in terms of "taking care of their own." Older people, for example, may feel duties toward their own younger family members but not necessarily toward those children who are strangers. This privatism is an understandable response, but a dangerous one. It can stimulate a backlash from the young, who in turn believe they owe nothing any longer to old people who are not members of their own families.

Most important perhaps, the fact that the elderly can, because of greater longevity combined with chronic illness, be dependent on others for longer periods of time than in the past introduces a new and troubling dimension to the morality of reciprocity: Even granting the existence of some fundamental duties, what are the boundaries? Which demands are excessive? At what point must the young, when their duties are in conflict, limit what they do for the old in order to meet the needs of their own children? Family members must simultaneously be dutiful parents to their own children and dutiful children to their own parents, and that combination can often be morally troubling in the extreme. It is important here to distinguish between intergenerational obligations (or obligation) within families and intergenerational obligations in society. Caring for older family members does not relieve the young of the duty to elderly people who are strangers to them but members of their society. There exists a duty to strangers as well, and thus the need to balance family and civic obligations.

A fresh cultural dialogue on intergenerational obligation in all its dimensions is crucial, with both the old and young taking part together. No longer can it be taken for granted that the moral traditions of reciprocity, which often functioned inadequately in any case, will command the kind of automatic respect they once did. We believe that the young have strong obligations to the old, and the old to the young. But how might that best be understood in the context of welfare programs designed to relieve the family of excessive burdens, and in the context of certain affectional and emotional needs that government can rarely meet in any case? Coping with these questions will require civic structures and mechanisms designed to facilitate a serious interchange between young and old. Adequate political and economic decisions cannot be made without a substrate of moral understanding well in place.

The most difficult problem will be that of balancing some different kinds of obligation: the obligations (1) of the old to their own welfare, (2) of government toward the old, and (3) of families toward their elderly members. While the dependency needs of the young can be demanding, medical progress creates a special problem with the old: are the young required to follow medical progress wherever it goes, providing through their taxes unlimited access to whatever technology will extend and improve the life of the old, whatever the cost, or will it be possible to discover or devise some natural or socially constructed limits?

Obligations or gratitude toward the old do not necessarily entail unlimited duties. The hard question is their scope and boundaries. This is sure to be a vexing problem for government in the future, where the scientific possibilities of providing medical benefit for the old can and probably will outrun the financial resources available to provide them. At what point can government obligations come to an end, throwing the problem back to families or to the elderly themselves? The question is complicated by clear evidence of a decline in the welfare state in the European countries; the effect of that development on the aged has yet to be charted. Realism requires that the problem of intergenerational obligation be seen in that context and its dimensions and implications factored into the moral and social equation.

Is it possible to determine some reasonable, minimal demands that every citizen can make on the state for health and welfare support? At the least, citizens can make a reasonable claim on government to help them avoid a premature death—that is, a death before age sixty-five or thereabouts, which for close to a century has been taken to be the conventional starting point for old age. But there is as yet no consensus about what can be demanded beyond that, or at what point the needs and desires of the old for their health and welfare must reasonably give way to other age groups. An intense public and political discussion will be needed on the scope and limits of health care for the elderly. This discussion will have to give careful attention to the importance of the family, but also its limitations in providing care. At its heart will be a moral problem of the first order: Just who, and in what way, is responsible for the elderly? How can we make certain that both young and old gain their fair share and that each helps to make possible the fair share of the other?

Recommendation 3. *An integrated set of priorities for young and old should be pursued as part of an effort to devise a fair and sensible allocation of resources between the generations and within the generations. The young and the old should work together to develop those priorities and be prepared to share equitably any limits on the use of resources that may be required.*

At no time have governments been able to provide all the social services or health care that the elderly might need, much less desire. Some degree of rationing, overt or covert, has been part of every health care system. Now, however, the need for restraining expenditures is all the more pronounced. Most governments have established policies to limit either specific budgets, or the percentage of the domestic national product devoted to health care, and usually both. Increasingly these limitations are cutting into the available services or shortly will. In that context, some kind of priority system will be necessary: What is comparatively more or less important to the health of the elderly? What priority should be given the health care needs of the elderly in comparison with the needs of other age groups?

On the latter question, we believe that the highest priority should be given to enhancing the possibility that young people will become old people, that is, to efforts to reduce premature death rates. If there are sufficient funds left after that end has been assured, then efforts to extend and improve the lives of the elderly are appropriate, though there are bound to be some limitations imposed at some point if health care budgets are in general limited.

In determining the needs of the elderly, the budget process should try to balance the needs for reduction of mortality and for acute-care medicine, on the one hand, and for long-term and home care needs, together with quality of life services, on the other. The imbalance between curing and caring, discussed above, is best dealt with in the budget process, where in the future available funds could be more sensibly distributed. A wise set of priorities would work to guarantee, first of all, good programs that provide primary and nursing care for the elderly, putting high-technology cure and the extension of life into a secondary position, at least until a good balance is achieved. Everyone is likely to need and benefit from services designed to provide care and comfort; that need will remain, and in that sense is fundamental, when the possibility of cure and the saving of life has passed. In that respect, the need for care is permanent, and that of life-extending medicine temporary, inherently limited by the failing bodies that are a part of aging and the boundaries set by the limitations of medical technology.

More generally, in setting overall priorities for the elderly in some countries, there is still an imperative need for an integration of welfare and health services, or at least their tight coordination. Priorities will be needed within integrated or coordinated budgets, a process made all the more difficult when different agencies and different procedures must be compared with each other. The division of services to the elderly into different budgets and budgeting processes is itself a sources of gaps in coverage and a failure to recognize how the different needs of the elderly are often all but indistinguishable from each other in their actual lives: poor housing can cause or exacerbate medical problems, for example, just as anxiety about social services can create mental-health problems. Ideally, then, welfare and health care budgets should become integrated into single budgets, but failing that, they should be developed together, recognizing that sharp lines are all but impossible to draw.

In setting social priorities, the most difficult discussion will require comparing the health and welfare needs of the old, where life and death may be at stake for them, and the welfare, educational, and social needs of the young. It will not be lives that are at stake for the young, but instead the quality and adequacy of those lives. Comparatively few high-technology interventions for the old, desperately needed on occasion, can consume resources that might otherwise be spent for preventive or rehabilitative services for other old people, or to improve significantly the educational opportunities of hundreds of children. How are such choices to be made, entailing as they do the comparison of incommensurable human goods? Despite their difficulty, means must be found to pursue such inquiries and to put them before the public, a public that must itself, young and old, be intimately a part of the debate.

Recommendation 4. *The burden upon women in the care of the elderly that has marked informal caregiving in the past cannot and should not be sustained. This change will require a new strategy in the division of responsibility for informal care and the development of new government programs to nourish caregiving of this kind.*

An important consequence of the changing ratio of young to old is a growing crisis in the ability of families to care for their elderly members. A combination of smaller families and a larger number of working women means that there are fewer and fewer people at home to provide care and companionship for the elderly. At the same time there is strong resistance to the unfair burden that traditional home care has placed upon women. To complicate the situation further, as governments are under new pressures to stabilize health care costs, programs to assist the elderly in living at home, either on their own or with their families, are at great risk. As these programs are undercut, the problem of care is thrown even more into the hands of families—and at just the time when they are increasingly unable to provide it.

This problem will not easily be solved, combining as it does external economic pressures and internal familial changes. Even if more money were available, that would not necessarily make much difference in the contemporary dynamics of the family; and even if families were better situated to care for their elderly, more money to help them do so would not easily be forthcoming. The problem, then, of finding an appropriate balance between the individual responsibility of the elderly for themselves and the responsibility of families and government for them is becoming especially acute.

One point seems clear: it will not be prudent in the future for the elderly or their families to depend too heavily, much less exclusively, on government to find a solution to the problem. Though increased expenditures, as we have argued, should go to such caring services as the elderly require, if the care-cure balance is to be corrected, that money will be hard to extract from government. New arrangements will be necessary and need to be advanced. Among them would be to devise fresh ways and new programs to make it easier for families to care for their elderly parents—ones less dependent upon women to provide the bulk of such care, or at least designed to reduce that burden if it cannot be avoided.

Among the possibilities here would be employment policies that are generous in allowing family members to stay home to assist elderly parents when needed, as is now often the case with child care for working parents. Of critical importance would be policies ensuring that those who do take time from their employment to provide care for an elderly family member are not professionally penalized for doing so. Subsidizing a part of the cost of hiring outside help could make a difference as well, as would generous policies of paid respite programs for family members. A much better training of physicians and other health care workers to counsel and work with families on the stress and tension of family care would make another significant contribution.

Inevitably perhaps, the elderly themselves may be forced to take a greater responsibility for their situation, when there is no other way to avoid that. It can be made clear, in a variety of ways, that people should look forward while still young to the day when they are old and will have to provide for themselves. In particular they should be educated to take seriously programs of preventive medicine to reduce the likelihood or early onset of crippling illness, disability, and frailty. The important scientific evidence about all the things the elderly can do to keep in good health—exercise, nutrition, and lifestyle generally, even when begun at a relatively late stage in life—should be widely disseminated. Most critically, perhaps, the elderly themselves can be much more effectively organized and motivated to care for each other. Various small and experimental programs in some countries have indicated the effectiveness of this approach.

As a matter of pure self-interest, the elderly should be helped to see that they may in the future have a stronger basis for solidarity with each other than with government; at the least, efforts to improve their mutual help could pay large dividends.

There will be no easy way to solve the problems now arising in the traditional heavy dependence upon families to care for their old. Government can help, as much with thoughtful programs as with money; and families, even as their possibilities for aiding the elderly decline, can be supported in many ways yet untried and given the benefits of both policies and public attitudes that will enable them to do decently well on limited resources.

> **Recommendation 5.** *Active efforts should be undertaken to help the elderly to organize politically and to define and articulate their major needs collectively. A high priority in that effort should be to end the frequent separation of health and welfare programs and to make clear to the public and government that no sharp or meaningful lines can be drawn between the varied and overlapping needs of the elderly: social, economic, and medical.*

Notably lacking in many countries is a conscious and sophisticated effort on the part of the elderly to organize themselves as a viable and potent political force. In the few countries where this course has been diligently pursued, the benefits have been striking: the elderly become a political power to be reckoned with, a point not lost on legislators. The elderly ought not, as a matter of sheer survival and in the interest of gaining their appropriate share of resources, leave themselves to the mercy of younger age-groups or to groups that do not have a strong representation of the elderly. The elderly themselves need to have ways politically and publicly to articulate their legitimate needs, to carry out research on their own behalf, and to have access to the political and cultural sources of power and influence in their country. This will be particularly important in those countries that have in the recent past depended exclusively upon the government for medical and welfare programs but that will now see power and prestige shared with newly emergent efforts at privatization. The elderly will now have some unparalleled opportunities to make their voice heard and will face some unparalleled hazards if they fail to do so.

Any significant effort on the part of the elderly, or their younger advocates, should encompass a number of closely coordinated activities. First and foremost among them, as mentioned above, would be a strong drive to integrate medical and social services, which in some countries are divided and uncoordinated. A reform of fixed-age retirement policies will be important in the future, not only to take account of the improved longevity and health of the elderly but also to help break down the too often rigid line between the employed and the nonemployed and allow part-time and flexible work opportunities even to those well advanced in years. An increase in programs to encourage the elderly to help and work with each other and to volunteer their services more widely is no less necessary.

In the Central European countries in particular, special efforts will be needed to overcome the lethargy and lack of political awareness induced by forty years of Communist domination. Those years saw political power and initiative removed from the people and placed exclusively in the hands of government. Not only did this disempower the elderly in making their needs known and publicly heard; it led to a passive dependence upon the state to look after their needs paternalistically. As it will be increasingly important in the future for the elderly to become more responsible for their own good health and to have a stronger, more central voice in the development of public policy, special education and political effort will be required in those countries. Since those countries are, moreover, engaged in some significant and far-reaching changes in their health care and social-welfare programs, it is vital that the elderly be a part of that reform process, not simply added on after the reform as a minor consideration.

In the end, no sharp line can be drawn between the meaning the elderly find for their own private lives and the role and dignity assigned them by society through the medium of its governmental programs and policies. They will reinforce and work in tandem with each other. The very effort to develop new programs for the elderly, which should involve the elderly themselves in a leading role, will strengthen their political self-consciousness while helping them simultaneously think through the possibilities for their own lives.

Recommendation 6. A public dialogue on the significance of old age in the common life of society should be advanced through educational programs, the media, and joint governmental-private efforts. These efforts should encompass future possibilities for the elderly in the realms of work and leisure. Additional efforts should be fostered to help the elderly think through their personal meanings and goals.

The starting point of a meaningful discussion of resource allocation to the elderly should be the place of the elderly both in society and in their own eyes. Who are these people to whom we want to allocate resources? Who are the elderly? What do we make of old age as a stage in life? Where do the elderly fit into the scheme of life devised, wittingly or unwittingly, by modern societies?

Every society has traditions and practices that affect the way the elderly think about themselves and the way they are thought about by others. The meaning of old age for individuals—what they make of their aging and how they come to value themselves—will be in part a function of the various messages society has conveyed to them in word and deed and of what the elderly themselves bring to their aging. The social significance of aging—the societal role assigned to the elderly and the public programs developed on their behalf—will not only influence the self-perception of the aged but also project a picture of the value placed upon them by society. From the latter picture will come most of the elements that determine, overtly or covertly, the amount and kind of resources made available to the elderly.

While every nation examined in our study has medical and welfare programs for the elderly in some form or other, there is a significant degree of variation from country to country in the quality and generosity of these programs. No less important, there is a significant variation in the self-perception by the elderly of their own value and that assigned them by their society. In some countries, good welfare and medical programs are matched by strong, often voluntary efforts to enhance and improve the dignity and public status of the elderly. In others, by contrast, poor governmental programs are matched by a public perception of the old as merely a burdensome problem, a view too often shared by the elderly themselves. In a few societies, strong government programs are not matched by a well-organized, politically effective cadre of the elderly; their lack of political force renders them vulnerable in the face of budget reductions, cut off from a direct voice in decisions crucial to them.

While retirement serves as a significant borderline in every country, some countries have begun substantial efforts to develop new roles and opportunities for the aged, while others have done almost nothing at all. In every country, however, there is an absence of a clear picture or positive image of the place of the elderly once their public work life has come to an end. Though they may live on for another two or three decades, few modern societies have creatively worked to make some rich and productive use of those added years. Retirement, for most, marks the end of the publicly valued role of an economic producer in the society. No alternative role has been developed to replace it. Without strenuous and focused efforts to develop such roles, it is all too easy for the elderly to feel themselves irrelevant and neglected, exactly the cultural status projected upon them.

A paradox in the life of individuals is that they must find their own personal meanings for life and death—for youth, adulthood, and old age— and yet they cannot well do this without the help of the larger community of which they are a part. Even in countries without a strong individualistic tradition, or where the value of solidarity is still prized, few societies any longer presume to instruct their citizens on how they should understand their own lives, a function once performed by religious traditions or homogeneous value systems. Historically, there is some evidence to suggest that those traditions and systems did help the elderly to make sense of their lives, usually by placing them in some larger context of religious, cultural, and generational transcendence.

Is it desirable to seek, once again, some degree of consensus on the meaning of old age for individual lives? Is it possible? The case against such an effort can seem compelling: in pluralistic societies, where the value of religious and philosophical freedom is prized, it is inappropriate, even hazardous, to seek for some common meaning. All too quickly a consensus on meaning can become an instrument of repression. Yet it is no less true that the secular citizens of modern societies find it extraordinarily hard to create personal meaning in a culture that does not allow, or encourage, its citizens to talk openly and comfortably with each other about the crucial phases of human life. Nor is it clear how government and other social institutions will come to prize and support the elderly if there seems to be a studied cultural indifference to the deeper issues that aging poses for the self-understanding of the old.

While there can, then, be dangers in a forced consensus, ways need to be developed that will permit public exchanges on the meaning of old age in the life cycle, and particularly an old age that is significantly longer for more and more people. This will not be easy to do. It will require the development of fresh cultural resources—such as media and educational programs—together with the shaping of a public language to talk about matters left of late to families or churches. It is most appropriate for private institutions to help the elderly develop their own sense of personal meaning in their lives. This is probably best done through informal but nonetheless organized programs that bring the elderly together to talk with each other about their lives and how they make sense of those lives. The simple sharing of their common stage in life with those in a like position can itself have a potent effect in clarifying for the elderly their own situation.

Concluding Reflections

The problems of health and welfare policies and programs for the old—those that will soon be upon us as well as those of the present—should be given the highest social and political priority. The remarkable ability of medicine to extend life has not been matched by a similar capacity to ensure a high level of health and individual flourishing. The gap is significant and is too often plugged by programs that cost more than we can afford and are probably in the long run unsustainable. Alternatively, the gap is plugged by programs of long-term institutional care and informal home care that are at worst inhumane and niggardly, and at best starved for adequate funds and well-trained health care workers and social workers.

The neglect of the emerging problems of health care for the elderly can in part be traced to the difficulty all democratic societies have in dealing with future problems; they too often get pushed aside in favor of more immediate crises. But there may also be in the case of health care and social services for the elderly a special fear of facing up early to concerns that promise to be especially wrenching, creating highly unpleasant and complex moral problems. They are coming and they are real. The longer they are put off, kept from the public eye, the more difficult they will be to handle when upon us. There is still time to set priorities, to examine and reexamine our traditional moral practices and conventions.

NOTE

This report is the outcome of a two-year research project entitled "Care for the Elderly: Goals, Resources, Priorities," organized jointly by The Institute for Bioethics, Maastricht, the Netherlands, and The Hastings Center, Briarcliff Manor, N.Y., USA. The research project members responsible for this volume represented eight countries in Western and Central Europe and North America. Their names and institutional affiliations are listed later in this book. In signing their names to the recommendations, the participants are indicating their general agreement with the project's conclusions, not necessarily all the details of the document. They also sign only on their own behalf and not on behalf of the governments or organizations for which they work. The 1993 European Year of the Elderly was a major stimulus for the research project.

Project Participants

W. Andrew Achenbaum is deputy director and professor of history at the Institute of Gerontology of the University of Michigan, Ann Arbor.

Gebhard Allert is a physician specializing in psychotherapy and a member of the medical faculty at the University of Ulm, Germany.

Bela Blasszauer is a lawyer and senior lecturer at the Medical University of Pécs in Pécs, Hungary.

Sarah-Vaughan Brakman is an assistant professor of philosophy at Villanova University, Villanova, Pennsylvania.

Daniel Callahan is president of The Hastings Center in Briarcliff Manor, New York.

Rob Houtepen is an associate professor in the Department of Health, Ethics, and Philosophy at the State University of Limburg in Maastricht, the Netherlands.

Bryan Jennett is emeritus professor of neurosurgery at the Institute of Neurological Sciences at the University of Glasgow, United Kingdom.

Malcolm Johnson is dean of the School of Health, Welfare, and Community Education at Open University in Milton Keynes, United Kingdom.

Harry R. Moody is deputy director of the Brookdale Center on Aging of Hunter College, New York, New York.

Ruud H. J. ter Meulen is Radboud Professor of Philosophy in the Department of Health Ethics of the State University of Limburg and senior researcher at the Institute for Bioethics, both in Maastricht, the Netherlands.

Mats Thorslund is a professor of social work and gerontology at Stockholm University, Stockholm, Sweden.

Eva Topinková is an assistant professor of geriatrics/gerontology at the Institute for Postgraduate Medicine in Prague, Czech Republic.

Index